# Study Guide to
# INTRODUCTORY PSYCHIATRY

## SECOND EDITION

A Companion to the
### *Introductory Textbook of Psychiatry,*
### Seventh Edition

# Study Guide to
# INTRODUCTORY
# PSYCHIATRY
## SECOND EDITION

A Companion to the
*Introductory Textbook of Psychiatry,*
**Seventh Edition**

Donald W. Black, M.D.

Professor Emeritus, University of Iowa Roy J. and
Lucille A. Carver College of Medicine, Iowa City, Iowa

Jordan Cates, M.D.

Staff Psychiatrist, Veterans Administration Medical Center;
Clinical Assistant Professor, Department of Psychiatry and Behavioral
Sciences, University of Oklahoma, Oklahoma City, Oklahoma

AMERICAN
**PSYCHIATRIC**
ASSOCIATION
**PUBLISHING**

If you wish to buy 50 or more copies of the same title, please go to www.appi.org/specialdiscounts for more information.

Second Edition

Manufactured in the United States of America on acid-free paper
25  24  23  22  21    5  4  3  2  1

American Psychiatric Association Publishing
800 Maine Avenue SW
Suite 900
Washington, DC 20024-2812
www.appi.org

# Contents

# PART II: ANSWER GUIDE

# Foreword

As most medical students have realized by now, studying as a pre–medical student in college and studying in medical school are usually very different things. Premedical students, like most undergraduates, "cram" for examinations with the goal of getting a good grade on the examination. Most of them don't care all that much about being able to remember the material in detail at some time in the future. In the language of cognitive science, they use "shallow encoding," while they would need to do "deep encoding" to retain and recall the information at a later time (e.g., in 5 or 10 years).

In medical school and residency, on the other hand, achieving deep encoding of learned materials is essential. Medical students are acquiring a treasure chest of knowledge that they will use for many years to come. A good physician is a person who has preserved masses of information on diverse topics and can organize and recall them when working with any patient who walks into his or her office. A primary care physician has perhaps the greatest challenge because of the need to diagnose and treat a diversity of diseases ranging from gastrointestinal to psychiatric. (And many problems that primary care physicians confront are psychiatric.) As one of my physician friends once said to me, "I can't be a primary care doctor because I'm not smart enough." There is a lot of truth in that statement—primary care doctors need to know *a lot*. But other specialties—cardiology, orthopedics, pediatrics—will also be called on to have good access not only to specialty knowledge but also to more general medical knowledge. You have to be "smart" to be any kind of physician.

So, what is the secret of achieving deep encoding? There are in fact many. Using this study guide will facilitate some of them. One secret is to go beyond rote memorization of information to accessing it and using it to answer questions. Another is to see how knowing a piece of information is consolidated when it is approached from several different directions—for example, diagnosis, treatment planning, and understanding disease mechanisms. This study guide will facilitate those examples and many more.

We owe a lot to my colleague and coauthor of the *Introductory Text-book of Psychiatry* and to his coauthor of this book for taking the time to write this study guide. They have taken painstaking care in thinking through the questions that students can answer after reading the various chapters of the textbook. When students answer a question correctly, it will help to consolidate their knowledge. When they miss a question, it will also help to consolidate, because they will need to figure out why they "got it wrong." Understanding and rectifying ignorance are as important as taking pride in having learned something well.

Donald Black has been a leader in psychiatric education for many years. He ran our residency program at University of Iowa with great success. He loves to teach and mentor students. He loves to see how residents can finish their training and go on to next steps—to private practice, to practice within a medical school, or to a postdoctoral fellowship in clinical care (e.g., geriatrics) or in a research environment (e.g., genetics and genomics, neuroimaging). He was fortunate to have had a highly talented resident, Jordan Cates, now in practice, help to create this wonderful study guide. Thank you, Don and Jordan!

*Nancy C. Andreasen, M.D., Ph.D.*
Andrew H. Woods Chair of Psychiatry and Director, Iowa Neuroimaging Consortium, University of Iowa Carver College of Medicine, Iowa City, Iowa

# Preface

Medical students, residents in psychiatry, and other learners have been enthusiastic about the *Introductory Textbook of Psychiatry* since it was first published in 1991. Now in its seventh edition, the book has changed and evolved as needed in order to stay current. After being urged to do so for many years, we wrote our first companion study guide for the sixth edition, now updated for compatibility with the seventh edition. This will give learners an opportunity to test their command of the knowledge of the material in the textbook. The questions are written to provide emphasis and clarity to major clinical issues.

We encourage readers to first answer the questions at the conclusion of each chapter in *Introductory Textbook of Psychiatry*, Seventh Edition, and then to use this study guide for additional and more detailed questions. The format replicates what might be encountered in specialty-certifying examinations. Each question is followed by multiple-choice responses, including plausible "distractors." The answer is then provided, with an explanation of the correct response as well as an explanation of why the other answers are incorrect. Each question is linked to a page or pages in the textbook.

We believe this guide has the potential to help readers gain a much greater understanding of the material. We hope you will find this study guide interesting and useful.

Although the guide and the many questions have been reviewed many times, it is possible that an incorrect response is included. If so, please feel free to contact the senior author at donald-black@uiowa.edu.

Good luck with your studies.

*Donald W. Black, M.D.*
*Jordan Cates, M.D.*

S T U D Y    G U I D E

**PART I**

# QUESTIONS

# CHAPTER 1

# Diagnosis and Classification

1.1 Which of the following terms is used to describe collections of symptoms that tend to co-occur and appear to have a characteristic course and outcome?

A. Disease.
B. Symptomatology.
C. Syndrome.
D. Pathophysiology.
E. Illness.

1.2 Which of the following is *not* a clinical reason to diagnose patients?

A. To reduce the complexity of clinical phenomena.
B. To provide the patient a label with which to identify.
C. To facilitate communication among clinicians.
D. To predict the course of illness.
E. To determine treatment options.

1.3 Which DSM edition first provided specific diagnostic criteria for mental disorders?

A. DSM-I.
B. DSM-II.
C. DSM-III.
D. DSM-IV.
E. DSM-5.

1.4 Which of the following is *not* an advantage of the DSM system?

A. It has substantially improved reliability of diagnoses.
B. It has substantially improved validity of diagnoses.
C. It has clarified the diagnostic process and history taking.
D. It has clarified and facilitated the process of differential diagnosis.
E. All the above are advantages of the DSM system.

1.5 You are asked to evaluate a 55-year-old man on a general medical floor. You determine that he is delirious because of a hepatic encephalopathy. You learn that he drinks large quantities of distilled spirits daily and smokes one pack of cigarettes per day. Considering the *International Classification of Diseases* (ICD) and DSM rules, how would you record his diagnoses (i.e., in order of importance)?

A. Delirium (principal diagnosis), alcohol use disorder, tobacco use disorder.
B. Delirium due to hepatic encephalopathy (principal diagnosis), alcohol use disorder, tobacco use disorder.
C. Alcohol use disorder (provisional diagnosis), delirium due to hepatic encephalopathy, tobacco use disorder.
D. Hepatic encephalopathy, delirium due to hepatic encephalopathy (principal diagnosis), alcohol use disorder, tobacco use disorder.
E. Delirium due to hepatic encephalopathy, hepatic encephalopathy, alcohol use disorder, tobacco use disorder.

1.6 You are evaluating a patient in the emergency department who you believe is likely experiencing a psychotic manic episode (bipolar I disorder with psychotic features). The patient is a poor historian, and you are not currently able to obtain collateral information to confirm the diagnosis. According to DSM, how should you document the diagnosis to reflect your uncertainty?

A. Rule out bipolar I disorder.
B. Evaluate for bipolar I disorder.
C. Bipolar I disorder versus psychosis not otherwise specified.
D. Bipolar I disorder (provisional).
E. Bipolar I disorder.

1.7   You are seeing a 25-year-old woman in the outpatient clinic for a routine follow-up visit. Major problems reported at the visit include stormy interpersonal relationships and frequent anger outbursts. You conclude that these symptoms result from her borderline personality disorder. The patient's symptoms also meet criteria for generalized anxiety disorder, and she smokes 10 cigarettes daily. How would you record the diagnoses according to DSM-5?

A. Axis I: generalized anxiety disorder, tobacco use disorder; Axis II: borderline personality disorder (principal diagnosis).
B. Borderline personality disorder (principal diagnosis), generalized anxiety disorder, tobacco use disorder.
C. Generalized anxiety disorder, borderline personality disorder, tobacco use disorder.
D. Tobacco use disorder, borderline personality disorder, generalized anxiety disorder.
E. Borderline personality disorder (provisional), generalized anxiety disorder, tobacco use disorder.

1.8   A 34-year-old woman comes to your office for new-onset depression. The history reveals that along with depression, she has developed cold intolerance, fatigue, and weight gain. Routine laboratory testing reveals hypothyroidism, which you believe is the cause of her depression. What is the correct way to record the diagnoses?

A. Major depressive disorder (principal diagnosis), hypothyroidism.
B. Depression due to hypothyroidism (principal diagnosis), hypothyroidism.
C. Hypothyroidism, depression due to hypothyroidism (provisional).
D. Hypothyroidism, depression due to hypothyroidism (principal diagnosis).
E. Hypothyroidism, major depressive disorder (principal diagnosis).

1.9   Which of the following is not included in DSM-5?

A. Comorbidity.
B. Diagnostic features.
C. Treatment guidelines.
D. Suicide risk.
E. Risk and prognostic factors.

# CHAPTER 2

# Interviewing and Assessment

2.1 A psychiatrist asks a patient to recall a list of three objects ("orange, airplane, tobacco") after 5 minutes. What type of memory does this test?

   A. Ultrashort-term memory.
   B. Very-short-term memory.
   C. Short-term memory.
   D. Medium-term memory.
   E. Long-term memory.

2.2 A psychiatrist asks a patient to tell her what the phrase "don't cry over spilled milk" means. The patient replies, "Milk isn't worth crying over because it's easy to come by." What does the patient's answer suggest?

   A. Illogicality.
   B. Poor abstraction.
   C. Derailment.
   D. Circumstantiality.
   E. Poverty of content of speech.

2.3 A man believes he is preventing cancer and maximizing his health by taking an expensive but otherwise innocuous herbal supplement. If asked, he will discuss the supplement with great interest but dismisses evidence that does not confirm his beliefs. Otherwise, this interest in the supplement has no significant influence on his day-to-day life. Which of the following terms best describes the man's beliefs?

A. Overvalued ideation.
B. Delusion.
C. Poor abstraction.
D. Impaired fund of knowledge.
E. Illogicality.

2.4 A patient admits to her psychiatrist that she sometimes worries that events she reads about in magazines indirectly comment on her personal life. For example, one of her favorite magazines had a recipe for banana cream pie, which made her think that somehow the editor knew that this was her favorite pie. The psychiatrist asks her if she really believes this, and the patient reports that sometimes it does seem "silly." What term best describes the woman's suspicion?

A. Illogicality.
B. Persecutory delusions.
C. Delusions of reference.
D. Ideas of reference.
E. Thought broadcasting.

2.5 A 35-year-old woman reports to her psychiatrist that, as part of a government conspiracy, a mind control device was implanted in her brain. She believes that the FBI (or possibly the CIA) is using this device to spy on her. Furthermore, she says that the device can control her body movements, making her feel like a puppet on a string. She describes how the device can remove thoughts from her brain like a vacuum cleaner while implanting thoughts that are not hers. Which of the following symptoms is *not* consistent with this patient's delusional system?

A. Delusions of passivity.
B. Thought withdrawal.
C. Thought insertion.
D. Somatic delusions.
E. Persecutory delusions.

2.6    A psychiatrist asks a patient where she lives. She replies, "I live in Springfield. It will be spring in another couple of months, but at least this winter has been mild. The winter tends to be pretty bad in Atlanta, which is where I lived until I moved to Springfield, but birds fly south in the winter. I'd really like to go to the beach just now." What is this an example of?

A. Tangentiality.
B. Circumstantiality.
C. Incoherence.
D. Illogicality.
E. Derailment.

2.7    A psychiatrist asks a patient if he enjoyed his own birthday party the prior week. The patient responds by laboriously describing preparations for the party and then going into minute detail about the party, including minutiae such as the order of arrival of the guests and vivid descriptions of the appetizers. Ten minutes into this story, the psychiatrist realizes that the patient has not yet answered his question. What is this an example of?

A. Circumstantiality.
B. Pressured speech.
C. Derailment.
D. Tangentiality.
E. Distractible speech.

2.8    A psychiatrist asks a patient where she lives. She replies, "I live in Springfield. The weather in spring makes me want to spring forth with joy. I like to drink fresh spring water. You need springs to build several different kinds of machines. Spring. Bring. Cling. Ring." What is the best way to describe this type of formal thought disorder?

A. Incoherence.
B. Clanging.
C. Distractible speech.
D. Pressured speech.
E. Alogia.

2.9    A psychiatrist is interviewing a manic patient. The patient speaks
       very rapidly, and it is very difficult for the psychiatrist to get a word
       in. The patient is unable to adequately answer many routine ques-
       tions because he is distracted by objects in the room such as chairs,
       the psychiatrist's identification badge, and the clock on the wall.
       Which of the following options best describes the patient's speech?

       A. Pressured speech.
       B. Distractible speech.
       C. Both pressured speech and distractible speech.
       D. Catatonic excitement.
       E. Circumstantiality.

2.10   In response to a routine question, a patient begins to answer
       appropriately but stops talking midsentence and stares off into
       space for 15 seconds. She then asks the interviewer to repeat the
       question. What does this exemplify?

       A. Poverty of speech.
       B. Poverty of content of speech.
       C. Circumstantiality.
       D. Perseveration.
       E. Thought blocking.

2.11   A psychiatrist asks a patient where she lives. She replies, "I lived
       in Springfield many years ago." What is the best way to describe
       this formal thought disorder?

       A. Tangentiality.
       B. Circumstantiality.
       C. Incoherence.
       D. Illogicality.
       E. Derailment.

2.12   A psychiatrist asks a patient where she lives. She replies, "I live
       in Springfield. In Springfield. That's where I live in Springfield."

       A. Tangentiality.
       B. Perseveration.
       C. Incoherence.
       D. Illogicality.
       E. Derailment.

2.13   A psychiatrist notes that a depressed patient is very slow to answer questions and that his speech and body movements are slow. Despite the slowness, the patient is fully aware of the situation and can answer questions appropriately. What is the correct term for this symptom?

A. Stupor.
B. Psychomotor retardation.
C. Psychomotor agitation.
D. Thought blocking.
E. Poverty of speech.

2.14   A patient reports to his psychiatrist that he has a fear of losing control and stabbing his 10-year-old son. He finds the thoughts very distressing. To ally his fears, he had his wife lock up all knives. What type of symptom has the man described to his doctor?

A. Specific phobia.
B. Delusion of guilt.
C. Compulsion.
D. Obsession.
E. Aggressive behavior.

# — CHAPTER 3 —

# Neurobiology and Genetics of Mental Illness

3.1   Which of the following is *not* a primary function of the prefrontal system?

A. Mediation of attention and perception.
B. Mediation of affect and emotion.
C. Fear processing.
D. Temporal sequencing of behavior.
E. Moral judgment.

3.2   Which of the following areas of the brain have a high concentration of dopamine $D_2$ receptors and may be important sites for antipsychotic drug action?

A. Locus coeruleus.
B. Caudate and putamen.
C. Raphe nuclei.
D. Nucleus basalis.
E. None of the above.

3.3   Which part of the brain is dedicated to speech production?

A. Broca's area.
B. Nucleus basalis.
C. Angular gyrus.
D. Wernicke's area.
E. Amygdala.

3.4 The nucleus accumbens is a key part of which functional system in the brain?

A. Prefrontal system.
B. Limbic system.
C. Memory system.
D. Attention system.
E. Reward system.

3.5 What is the primary neurotransmitter in the brain reward system, which is also associated with adventuresome and exploratory behaviors?

A. Dopamine.
B. Norepinephrine.
C. γ-Aminobutyric acid (GABA).
D. Serotonin.
E. Glutamate.

3.6 Where does the brain's noradrenergic system originate?

A. Raphe nuclei.
B. Hypothalamus.
C. Ventral tegmental area.
D. Locus coeruleus.
E. Nucleus accumbens.

3.7 Which of the following nuclei in the brain contain the cell bodies of an important group of acetylcholine neurons?

A. Nucleus basalis.
B. Locus coeruleus.
C. Raphe nuclei.
D. Substantia nigra.
E. Caudate nucleus.

3.8 Which neurotransmitter regulates arousal, wakefulness, and appetite?

A. Histamine.
B. Acetylcholine.
C. Dopamine.

D. Orexin.

E. Glutamate.

3.9 Family studies of mental illness have shown that most major mental illnesses "run in families." Which of the following is *not* an essential element of a family study?

A. Identifying people with the disorder of interest (e.g., schizophrenia).

B. Identifying people who can serve as control subjects.

C. Interviewing first-degree relatives of ill persons and control subjects.

D. Comparing rates of the disorder of interest in relatives of those with the mental illness in question and relatives of control subjects.

E. Showing that the illness has a definitive genetic component.

3.10 Which type of study applies statistical analyses to large databases containing DNA from thousands of individuals affected by specific disorders?

A. Linkage study.

B. Candidate gene study.

C. Genome-wide association study (GWAS).

D. Copy number variant survey.

E. Microarray analysis.

3.11 Which of the following statements accurately characterizes DNA methylation?

A. DNA methylation alters the genome. Methyl groups are added to segments of DNA, turning genes on.

B. DNA methylation alters the genome. Methyl groups are added to segments of DNA, turning genes off.

C. DNA methylation does not alter the genome. Methyl groups are added to segments of DNA, turning genes on.

D. DNA methylation does not alter the genome. Methyl groups are added to segments of DNA, turning genes off.

E. None of the above.

# — CHAPTER 4 —

# Neurodevelopmental (Child) Disorders

4.1    What is the standard test used to assess the intelligence of children between ages 6 and 16 years?

A. Stanford-Binet Intelligence Scale.
B. Wechsler Intelligence Scale for Children—Fifth Edition (WISC-V).
C. Weschler Individual Achievement Test.
D. Kaufman Assessment Battery for Children.
E. Wechsler Preschool and Primary Scale of Intelligence.

4.2    Intellectual disabilities are characterized by which of the following?

A. IQ measured to be at least two standard deviations below the mean and deficits in adaptive functioning.
B. Deficits in intellectual functions without regard to adaptive functioning.
C. Deficits in intellectual functions and deficits in adaptive functioning.
D. Deficits in adaptive functioning without regard to intellectual functions.
E. IQ measured to be at least three standard deviations below the mean regardless of deficits in adaptive functioning.

4.3    What is the most common heritable cause of intellectual disability?

A. Down syndrome.
B. Fragile X syndrome.
C. Tay-Sachs disease.

D. Prader-Willi syndrome.

E. Williams syndrome.

4.4 A 25-year-old man with intellectual disability has lived in a group home throughout his adult life. He can read his name and a few other words. He can take care of his activities of daily living such as bathing and other personal hygiene tasks and doing laundry. He was in special education classes throughout school. What is the probable severity of his intellectual disability?

A. Mild.

B. Moderate.

C. Severe.

D. Profound.

E. Unable to estimate.

4.5 A mother of an 8-year-old girl asks her family doctor what she can do about her child's speech impediment. The girl displays frequent repetitions or prolongations of sounds, often pauses in the middle of a word, and frequently fills her speech with "um" or "like," which she then repeats ("um-um-um"). Which of the following is the girl's most likely communication disorder?

A. Language disorder.

B. Speech sound disorder.

C. Childhood-onset fluency disorder.

D. Social (pragmatic) communication disorder.

E. Autism spectrum disorder.

4.6 An 8-year-old boy is brought to a child psychiatrist for an evaluation. His parents report that he is socially awkward and has trouble making friends, but his grades have always been good. The boy is polite but overly formal in conversation. He avoids eye contact. His parents report that he sticks to a rigid routine at home and has an unusually intense interest in U.S. presidents and can name all of them in correct order. When this topic is brought up, the boy begins a lengthy discourse on them. Which of the following is the best diagnosis?

A. Language disorder.

B. Speech sound disorder.

C. Childhood-onset fluency disorder.

D. Social (pragmatic) communication disorder.

E. Autism spectrum disorder.

4.7    Treatment with stimulant medications in children with attention-deficit/hyperactivity disorder (ADHD)...

A. Increases risk for later substance abuse.

B. Decreases risk for later substance abuse.

C. Does not affect risk for substance abuse.

D. Is associated with a worse long-term outcome of ADHD.

E. Increases risk for abuse of stimulant medications only.

4.8    What is the prevalence of ADHD in children?

A. 1%–2%.

B. 5%.

C. 10%.

D. 20%.

E. >30%.

4.9    A 9-year-old boy is brought to his pediatrician by his parents, who are concerned about the possibility of ADHD. His teacher says that he is frequently in trouble for fighting with other children and that he refuses to obey classroom rules. He frequently steals small items from his peers and the school cafeteria. He also talks out of turn and has trouble staying in his seat. His parents report that he has lots of energy and that he "bounces off the walls" at home. He talks back to his parents. Which of the following symptoms in this case is most suggestive of ADHD?

A. Fighting with other children.

B. Refusal to obey classroom rules.

C. Stealing.

D. Talking back to parents.

E. Difficulty staying in his seat.

4.10   The pediatrician caring for the boy described in the previous vignette (4.9) has decided to prescribe medication to target ADHD. Which of the following response options is considered a first-line treatment?

A. Guanfacine.

B. Methylphenidate.

C. Clonidine.

D. Risperidone.

E. Atomoxetine.

4.11 Which of the following is *not* a common side effect of the stimulant medications commonly used to treat ADHD?

A. Weight gain.

B. Insomnia.

C. Stomach upset.

D. Irritability.

E. Appetite suppression.

4.12 A 9-year-old boy of average intelligence is making satisfactory grades in all subjects in school except math, which he is failing. His Iowa Test of Basic Skills score confirms satisfactory performance on all subjects except math, which is considerably lower than average. He sometimes shows irritation and frustration in the classroom during math class, but his behavior is otherwise unremarkable. His parents do not have concerns about his mood or behavior at home. Which of the following response options will be most beneficial for this child?

A. Remedial instruction in math and instruction in compensatory learning strategies.

B. Methylphenidate.

C. Fluoxetine.

D. Atomoxetine.

E. Cognitive-behavioral therapy.

4.13 Which of the following response options is *not* considered a stereotypic movement when considering the diagnosis of stereotypic movement disorder?

A. Head banging.

B. Rocking.

C. Hitting one's own body.

D. Nonrhythmic, jerky movements of the neck.

E. Hand waving.

4.14  How does the diagnosis of Tourette's disorder differ from a persistent motor or vocal tic disorder?

  A. Patients with Tourette's disorder have coprolalia (offensive vocal tics).
  B. Tics in Tourette's disorder are of longer duration than tics that occur in motor or vocal tic disorder.
  C. Patients with Tourette's disorder have both motor and vocal tics.
  D. Tourette's disorder is associated with streptococcal infection.
  E. Tourette's disorder has high comorbidity with obsessive-compulsive disorder.

4.15  Which of the following medications are FDA approved to treat pediatric depression?

  A. Fluoxetine and escitalopram.
  B. Citalopram and paroxetine.
  C. Venlafaxine and nefazodone.
  D. Sertraline and citalopram.
  E. Escitalopram and citalopram.

# CHAPTER 5

# Schizophrenia Spectrum and Other Psychotic Disorders

5.1 Which of the following statements *mischaracterizes* schizophrenia?

A. Patients have a "split" personality.
B. Patients have disability in their capacity to think clearly.
C. Patients have disability in their capacity to experience normal emotions.
D. Patients typically develop symptoms in early adulthood.
E. Patients often develop bizarre hallucinations and delusions.

5.2 A 45-year-old man has sought help for "stress." He attributes his stress to what he believes is a conspiracy by coworkers to get him fired by "arranging" work-related incidents that reflect poorly on him, such as hiding reports he's written or stealing needed documents. He has threatened to sue the coworkers, who have denied the allegations. As his psychiatrist, you find yourself unable to get him to talk about other issues. He has no auditory or visual hallucinations or any history of a mood disorder. His dress and grooming are appropriate, and his thoughts are well organized. Which of the following is the most likely diagnosis?

A. Schizophrenia.
B. Schizoaffective disorder.
C. Schizophreniform disorder.

D. Delusional disorder.

E. Bipolar I disorder.

5.3 At what age do women typically develop schizophrenia?

A. 13–18 years.

B. 18–25 years.

C. 21–30 years.

D. 35–50 years.

E. >50 years.

5.4 Which of the following is an example of a "first-rank" symptom of schizophrenia as identified by psychiatrist Kurt Schneider?

A. The patient believes that thoughts are being inserted into his or her mind.

B. The patient believes that the government is spying on him or her.

C. The patient believes that his or her masturbation has led to insanity.

D. The patient believes the somatic delusion that his or her heart has stopped beating.

E. The patient experiences the tactile hallucination that insects are crawling under his or her skin.

5.5 You are evaluating a 30-year-old woman with schizophrenia admitted to a psychiatric inpatient unit. She believes that she is dead and no longer exists. She will not accept any evidence to the contrary. What type of delusion is this?

A. Persecutory delusion.

B. Grandiose delusion.

C. Nihilistic delusion.

D. Somatic delusion.

E. Religious delusion.

5.6 Which phase of schizophrenia is characterized by subtle behavior changes that include social withdrawal, work impairment, blunting of emotion, avolition, and odd ideas and behavior?

A. Prodromal phase.

B. Active phase.

C. Residual phase.
D. Cataleptic phase.
E. Schizoaffective phase.

5.7    You are treating a patient with schizophrenia on a psychiatric in-
       patient unit. The patient has displayed disorganized thinking
       and behavior throughout hospitalization, such as tangential
       speech and dressing in a bizarre manner. One day at morning
       rounds, the patient mimics your hand gestures without explana-
       tion. What is the term for this behavior?

       A. Echolalia.
       B. Echopraxia.
       C. Catatonic stupor.
       D. Negativism.
       E. Stereotypy.

5.8    A 20-year-old man with schizophrenia comes to your clinic for a
       scheduled follow-up visit, accompanied by his mother, with
       whom he lives. His disorder is well controlled with a second-
       generation antipsychotic. He reports mild auditory hallucina-
       tions but is not bothered by them. His mother is concerned that
       her son is inactive much of the day and must be prompted to
       groom himself. He prefers to watch TV all day without engaging
       in any other activities. The patient shows some affective blunting
       but has not had depressive or manic symptoms during his ill-
       ness. He reports restful sleep and has a healthy appetite. He tol-
       erates his medication without noticeable adverse effects and says
       he feels "pretty good" about his current situation. How should
       you address the mother's concerns?

       A. Prescribe a stimulant to increase his energy.
       B. Prescribe an antidepressant to treat his negative symptoms.
       C. Reassess the patient for schizoaffective disorder and consider
          adding a mood stabilizer.
       D. Reduce the dose of the antipsychotic.
       E. Provide psychoeducation to the patient's mother.

5.9    A 24-year-old woman is admitted to an inpatient psychiatric unit
       for acute psychosis. She endorses auditory hallucinations and
       persecutory delusions and has an inappropriate affect. She has
       had no previous episodes and has not abused substances, and a

medical workup is negative. She has not had symptoms of depression or mania. At this point, her total duration of illness is 2 weeks. Which of the following is the best diagnosis?

A. Schizophrenia.
B. Schizoaffective disorder.
C. Schizophreniform disorder.
D. Brief psychotic disorder.
E. Bipolar disorder.

5.10  Peripartum onset is a specifier for which DSM-5 psychotic disorder?

A. Schizophrenia.
B. Schizoaffective disorder.
C. Schizophreniform disorder.
D. Brief psychotic disorder.
E. Bipolar disorder.

5.11  A 24-year-old woman is admitted to an inpatient psychiatric unit after developing a recurrence of psychotic symptoms in the setting of medication noncompliance. She hears voices telling her not to take her medication and thinks her psychiatrist is poisoning her. For that reason, she stopped taking her antipsychotic 2 weeks earlier. She denies abusing substances, and a urine drug screen is negative. There are no clear symptoms of depression or of mania. Two months earlier, she experienced her first psychotic episode, which lasted for 3 weeks but resolved with antipsychotic medication. Which of the following is the best diagnosis?

A. Schizophrenia.
B. Schizoaffective disorder.
C. Schizophreniform disorder.
D. Brief psychotic disorder.
E. Bipolar disorder.

5.12  Which of the following risk factors is associated with poor outcome in schizophrenia?

A. Female gender.
B. Insidious onset of symptoms.
C. Short prodrome.
D. Married or partnered.
E. Later onset.

5.13 Which of the following brain abnormalities in schizophrenia is associated with poor premorbid functioning, negative symptoms, poor response to treatment, and cognitive impairment?

A. Sulcal enlargement.
B. Cerebellar atrophy.
C. Decreased size of frontal lobe.
D. Ventricular enlargement.
E. Decreased size of thalamus.

5.14 Which of the following individuals has the lowest risk for developing schizophrenia?

A. Sibling of a person with schizophrenia.
B. Member of the general population.
C. Identical twin of a person with schizophrenia.
D. Nonidentical twin of a person with schizophrenia.
E. Child having one parent with schizophrenia.

5.15 A 30-year-old woman with auditory hallucinations and persecutory delusions is admitted to an inpatient psychiatric unit after developing euphoria, insomnia, agitation, and pressured speech. Her psychotic symptoms are usually well controlled with risperidone, a second-generation antipsychotic. She has a history of major depressive episodes, but she has psychotic symptoms even after the episodes resolve. What is the usual treatment for her disorder?

A. Switch to clozapine from risperidone.
B. Add lithium or valproate to the risperidone.
C. Start a selective serotonin reuptake inhibitor (SSRI) antidepressant.
D. Add the first-generation antipsychotic haloperidol to the risperidone.
E. Add the benzodiazepine clonazepam to the risperidone.

5.16 Which of the following mechanisms of action has been hypothesized to explain the effectiveness of antipsychotic medications?

A. Dopamine ($D_2$) receptor blockade.
B. 5-Hydroxytryptamine (serotonin) type 2 receptor (5-$HT_2$) blockade.

C. Glutamate receptor blockade.

D. Inhibition of serotonin reuptake.

E. Inhibition of dopamine reuptake.

5.17 Which of the following psychosocial treatments has been shown to reduce rates of relapse in schizophrenia?

A. Cognitive-behavioral therapy.

B. Interpersonal psychotherapy.

C. Social skills training.

D. Family therapy.

E. Vocational rehabilitation.

5.18 Which of the following response options is consistent with a diagnosis of schizoaffective disorder but not major depression or bipolar disorder?

A. Manic episodes accompanied by hallucinations and delusions.

B. Depressive episodes accompanied by hallucinations and delusions.

C. Hallucinations and delusions for at least 2 weeks in the absence of a major mood episode.

D. Presence of a mixed mood episode accompanied by hallucinations and delusions.

E. Symptoms of a major mood episode present for 25% of the total duration of the illness.

# CHAPTER 6

# Mood Disorders

6.1 Who first differentiated bipolar disorder from schizophrenia?

A. Eugen Bleuler.
B. Emil Kraepelin.
C. Sigmund Freud.
D. Kurt Schneider.
E. Carl Jung.

6.2 What is the minimum duration of a manic episode?

A. 12 hours.
B. 1–2 days.
C. 4 days.
D. 7 days.
E. 2 weeks.

6.3 Which of the following features is consistent with a hypomanic episode but *not* a manic episode?

A. Presence of hallucinations and delusions.
B. Duration of at least 1 week.
C. Elevated mood.
D. Decreased need for sleep.
E. Lack of marked social and occupational dysfunction.

6.4 A 28-year-old man is brought to the emergency department by the police for a psychiatric evaluation after his neighbors reported that he was behaving erratically. He is irritable with pressured speech and has slept only a few hours in the past several days. He believes that the FBI has implanted a microchip in his brain to record his thoughts and send him messages. He has been spending several hours each day making blueprints for lethal booby traps for his home to protect himself against government agents. He derails frequently in conversation. His physical examination is significant for dental caries, and his urine drug screen is positive for amphetamines. Why would it be premature to diagnose this patient with bipolar I disorder based on this presentation?

A. Presence of psychosis.
B. Persecutory delusions.
C. Mood is irritable rather than elevated.
D. Amphetamines present in drug screen.
E. Lack of grandiosity.

6.5　A 10-year-old boy is brought to his family physician by his parents. He has had recurrent severe behavioral outbursts at home and at school several times a week for the past several years. Outbursts are typically in reaction to minor disappointments or when he is asked to do routine chores. His parents did not seek attention for this problem because they thought he would outgrow it. Between outbursts, the boy's mood is "grumpy." Which of the following is the most likely diagnosis?

A. Disruptive mood dysregulation disorder.
B. Bipolar II disorder.
C. Major depressive disorder.
D. Persistent depressive disorder.
E. Unspecified depressive disorder.

6.6　A 35-year-old woman comes to your clinic to establish care. She reports that she has been depressed since adolescence with ongoing symptoms of low mood throughout the day, feelings of worthlessness, and low energy. She does not remember any recent period in the past several years that she was free of depression. Which of the following is the best diagnosis?

A. Major depressive disorder.
B. Persistent depressive disorder.
C. Disruptive mood dysregulation disorder.
D. Unspecified depressive disorder.
E. Bipolar II disorder.

6.7　A 30-year-old man comes to your clinic seeking help for depression. He reports feeling depressed most of each day for the past 3 weeks. He complains of poor sleep, low energy, inability to concentrate, and diminished appetite. He has lost interest in his work, and he spends much of his time watching TV. He has lost 5 pounds. He has had thoughts of hanging himself but does not think he would actually try to kill himself because of responsibility to his family. This is his fourth episode of depression since adolescence, and he has no history of mania or hypomania. Previous episodes have resolved spontaneously within a few months, and he is symptom free between episodes. Which of the following is the best diagnosis?

A. Disruptive mood dysregulation disorder.
B. Bipolar I disorder.
C. Major depressive disorder.
D. Persistent depressive disorder.
E. Unspecified depressive disorder.

6.8　A 60-year-old woman develops depressive symptoms following the death of her husband 1 month earlier. She reports trouble sleeping, feelings of guilt, low energy, and decreased appetite. She has difficulty paying attention to conversations with friends. She has thoughts about wanting to go to sleep and not wake up, thereby "joining" her deceased husband. When explored, it turns out that the patient's guilty feelings related to not telling her husband how much he was loved. The patient denies previous episodes of depression. Which of the following is the best diagnosis?

A. Bereavement.
B. Major depressive disorder.
C. Unspecified depressive disorder.
D. Persistent depressive disorder.
E. Bipolar II disorder.

6.9　What does it mean for a patient with bipolar disorder to have "rapid-cycling"?

A. Severe mood swings throughout the day.
B. Switching between mania and depression several times throughout a week.

C. At least four distinct mood episodes (e.g., mania, depression) in 1 year.

D. At least four distinct mood episodes (e.g., mania, depression) in 1 month.

E. None of the above.

6.10  A major depressive episode characterized by interpersonal rejection sensitivity, increased appetite, and hypersomnia indicates the presence of which of the following specifiers?

A. Atypical features.

B. Melancholic features.

C. Catatonic features.

D. Diurnal variation.

E. None of the above.

6.11  What is the lifetime prevalence for major depression?

A. 3%.

B. 10%.

C. 17%.

D. 38%.

E. >50%.

6.12  Major depressive disorder has been associated with all the following pathophysiological abnormalities *except*

A. Increased rapid eye movement (REM) sleep latency.

B. Volumetric reductions of subgenual prefrontal cortex.

C. Decreased slow-wave sleep.

D. Blunting of growth hormone output in response to insulin challenge.

E. Abnormal suppression of cortisol following dexamethasone administration.

6.13  Which of the following medications is *least* appropriate for the treatment of acute mania?

A. Carbamazepine.

B. Lithium.

C. Second-generation antipsychotic.

D. Gabapentin.

E. Valproate.

6.14    Which of the following is a first-line treatment for depression?

   A. Second-generation antipsychotic.
   B. Selective serotonin reuptake inhibitor (SSRI).
   C. Tricyclic antidepressant.
   D. Monoamine oxidase inhibitor (MAOI).
   E. Intranasal ketamine.

6.15    Brexanolone can be used to treat which of the following?

   A. Disruptive mood dysregulation disorder.
   B. Postpartum depression.
   C. Major depressive disorder.
   D. Bipolar I disorder.
   E. Schizoaffective disorder.

6.16    A 30-year-old man with major depressive disorder has not re-
        sponded to several trials of antidepressants. His insurer has ap-
        proved the use of intranasal esketamine, which is FDA approved
        for treatment-refractory depression. Which of the following side
        effects could your patient experience from the use of the drug?

   A. Dissociation.
   B. Memory impairment.
   C. Nausea and vomiting.
   D. Scalp discomfort.
   E. Hoarseness and cough.

# — CHAPTER 7 —

# Anxiety Disorders

7.1   A 7-year-old girl is brought to a therapist by her parents because she refuses to attend school. She has pretended to be sick ("Mommy, my tummy hurts") several times a week for the past month to avoid going to school. She reports fear of being away from her mother during the day and has nightmares of "bad accidents" happening to her mother. Which of the following is the most likely diagnosis?

   A. Generalized anxiety disorder.
   B. Social anxiety disorder.
   C. Separation anxiety disorder.
   D. Panic disorder.
   E. Specific phobia.

7.2   A teacher asks the parents of a 10-year-old boy to meet with her. She reports that since the boy started at the school 2 months ago, he has barely said a word and participates minimally in classroom activities. The parents report that, on the contrary, the boy is very talkative at home, and they haven't noticed any areas of concern. Which of the following is the most likely diagnosis?

   A. Generalized anxiety disorder.
   B. Social anxiety disorder.
   C. Separation anxiety disorder.
   D. Selective mutism.
   E. Specific phobia.

7.3   What is the primary fear that underlies social anxiety disorder?

   A. Social situations.
   B. Intimacy.

C. Sexual inadequacy.

D. Public humiliation.

E. Narcissistic injury.

7.4 What is the typical age at onset for social anxiety disorder?

A. Preschool years.

B. Elementary school age.

C. Adolescence.

D. Early adulthood.

E. Middle adulthood.

7.5 All but which of the following medication classes is effective in treating social anxiety disorder?

A. Selective serotonin reuptake inhibitors (SSRIs).

B. Monoamine oxidase inhibitors (MAOIs).

C. Tricyclic antidepressants (TCAs).

D. β-Blockers.

E. Benzodiazepines.

7.6 A 24-year-old woman presents to the emergency department complaining of the sudden onset of shortness of breath, dizziness, diaphoresis, chest pain, and a sense of impending doom. Her medical workup is negative, and her symptoms resolve within 30 minutes. She has had multiple previous episodes and fears her next spell. She avoids public places for fear of having an episode in public. Which of the following is the most likely diagnosis?

A. Generalized anxiety disorder.

B. Specific phobia.

C. Panic disorder.

D. Separation anxiety disorder.

E. Social anxiety disorder.

7.7 Which of the following medications is the best long-term treatment option for specific phobia?

A. Fluoxetine.

B. Lorazepam.

C. Sertraline.

D. Alprazolam.

E. None of the above.

7.8 Which two psychiatric disorders are the most likely to be comorbid with panic disorder?

A. Generalized anxiety disorder and major depressive disorder.

B. Generalized anxiety disorder and social anxiety disorder.

C. Major depressive disorder and alcohol use disorder.

D. Specific phobia and alcohol use disorder.

E. Persistent depressive disorder and generalized anxiety disorder.

7.9 What substance has been implicated in the "false suffocation alarm" theory of panic disorder?

A. Carbon dioxide ($CO_2$).

B. Oxygen.

C. Sodium lactate.

D. Melatonin.

E. Carbon monoxide.

7.10 A 20-year-old college student develops symptoms of intense anxiety, racing heart, dizziness, diaphoresis, and shortness of breath. The symptoms resolve within less than 30 minutes. Prior to developing these symptoms, he had consumed several cups of coffee to help him stay up late to study for an examination. He has had no previous episodes. Which of the following is the most likely diagnosis?

A. Panic disorder.

B. Specific phobia.

C. Social phobia.

D. Substance-induced anxiety disorder.

E. Generalized anxiety disorder.

7.11 What is the literal meaning of the term *agoraphobia*?

A. Fear of people.

B. Fear of crowds.

C. Fear of open spaces.

D. Fear of the marketplace.

E. Fear of enclosed spaces.

7.12   A 30-year-old woman is meeting with her new family physician and reports feeling "wound up" all the time. She describes herself as a "worrier" and feels like she has always been this way. She tends to worry and ruminate about everything ("my health, my husband's health, our finances") but also reports insomnia and muscle tension in her neck and shoulders. She has a hard time concentrating. She drinks one cup of coffee in the morning but otherwise does not use stimulants. She denies being depressed or using alcohol or street drugs. Which of the following is the most likely diagnosis?

A. Separation anxiety disorder.
B. Generalized anxiety disorder.
C. Substance-induced anxiety disorder.
D. Agoraphobia.
E. Panic disorder.

7.13   Which of the following medications can be effective in treating generalized anxiety disorder in addition to individual psychotherapy?

A. Buspirone.
B. Escitalopram.
C. Venlafaxine.
D. Duloxetine.
E. All the above.

# —— CHAPTER 8 ——

# Obsessive-Compulsive and Related Disorders

8.1 Which of the following is *not* considered an obsession according to DSM-5?

A. Recurrent concerns about germs or contamination.
B. Fixation on the appearance of a particular body part.
C. Intrusive and disturbing thoughts about a loved one being murdered.
D. Obsessive desire to achieve ambitious career goals.
E. Need to collect worthless items and being unable to throw things away.

8.2 Which of the following behaviors is *not* considered a compulsive ritual?

A. Handwashing.
B. Counting.
C. Gambling.
D. Checking.
E. Symmetrical arranging.

8.3 A 34-year-old man with generalized anxiety disorder tells his psychiatrist that he is worried that he may have OCD after reading an article on the Internet. He checks his door locks several times each morning before leaving for work, but this has never made him late for work. He worries that burglars could enter the house, but he is able to put the thought out of his mind after leaving his home. He has had these behaviors since adolescence.

There is no family history of OCD. Based on this information, what should the psychiatrist tell this patient?

A. "We should start clomipramine immediately to target your OCD."
B. "OCD is not likely, based on the age at onset of your symptoms."
C. "OCD is not likely, based on your negative family history."
D. "OCD is not likely because your symptoms are so mild."
E. "OCD is not likely, based on your established diagnosis of generalized anxiety disorder."

8.4   A 25-year-old man sees a psychiatrist for help with his OCD. He spends 2–3 hours each day arranging his bookshelves at home and is fed up with his need to do this. He feels that he is unable to stop his behavior and is afraid to have people over to his home for fear they might "mess up" the shelves. He has never sought treatment because he thought that he could handle it on his own. Which of the following is the best treatment strategy for this patient?

A. Clomipramine.
B. Fluoxetine.
C. Cognitive-behavioral therapy.
D. Fluoxetine plus cognitive-behavioral therapy.
E. Family therapy.

8.5   A patient presents to establish care with a new psychiatrist for treatment of OCD. He has seen several psychiatrists and therapists in the past 10 years, but he is frustrated because none of the treatments has been curative. How should the psychiatrist respond to this patient's concern?

A. Review the patient's adherence to specific medications.
B. Ask how long the patient has been able to stay in exposure therapy.
C. Recommend a new medication.
D. Inform the patient that OCD tends to be chronic.
E. None of the above.

8.6   Which of the following disorders appears to be genetically linked with OCD?

A. Pediatric autoimmune neuropsychiatric disorders associated with streptococcal infections (PANDAS).

B. Tourette's disorder.

C. Epilepsy.

D. Huntington's disease.

E. Sydenham's chorea.

8.7    A 17-year-old girl is brought to a psychiatrist by her concerned parents. She spends significant amounts of time staring at her nose in the mirror and has been saving her money for a rhinoplasty. The patient says that her nose is ugly and that her classmates stare at it, making fun of her through coded references. She cannot be reassured by her family that her nose looks normal and is even attractive. On examination, the nose appears unremarkable. She reports feeling demoralized by her concerns about her nose but has no history of depression, and she is not psychotic. There is no evidence of a thought disorder. Which of the following is the best diagnosis?

A. OCD with somatic obsessions.

B. Obsessive-compulsive personality disorder.

C. Delusional disorder, somatic type.

D. Body dysmorphic disorder.

E. Schizophrenia.

8.8    A 30-year-old man sees a psychiatrist at his wife's insistence. She is concerned about the possibility of him having OCD after watching a TV show about hoarding. He has an extensive video game collection that he started at age 7. His collection is neatly arranged on shelves that do not take up much space. He is proud of his collection, and he would never think about getting rid of a single title because he sees no reason to do so. He enjoys playing video games for an hour or so each day, but otherwise keeps busy with work. He is tight with money and insists on doing many household chores himself because he believes that his family can never do the chores to his exacting standards. He has rigid political views that he happily shares with others on a social networking site. He does not feel that he has a significant problem with depression or anxiety. Which of the following is the most likely diagnosis?

A. OCD.

B. Obsessive-compulsive personality disorder.

C. Hoarding disorder.

D. Internet gaming disorder.

E. Marital discord (e.g., partner-relational problem).

8.9    What kind of psychotherapy is recommended for trichotillomania?

A. Supportive psychotherapy.

B. Habit reversal therapy.

C. Psychodynamic psychotherapy.

D. Interpersonal psychotherapy.

E. Acceptance and commitment therapy.

8.10    Which tricyclic antidepressant has shown benefit for trichotillomania?

A. Imipramine.

B. Doxepin.

C. Clomipramine.

D. Amitriptyline.

E. Nortriptyline.

8.11    A 31-year-old woman has many open and bleeding sores on her forearms. She has sought help from dermatologists, who have prescribed various creams, all to no avail. The last dermatologist insisted that the woman seek a psychiatric evaluation. Which of the following is the most likely diagnosis?

A. Trichotillomania.

B. Unspecified obsessive-compulsive and related disorder.

C. Excoriation disorder.

D. Delusional disorder, somatic type.

E. OCD.

8.12    In excoriation disorder, what is the most common site for skin picking?

A. Face.

B. Hands.

C. Feet.

D. Arms.

E. Torso.

# — CHAPTER 9 —

# Trauma- and Stressor-Related Disorders

9.1    A 7-year-old boy is brought to a child psychiatrist by his new fos-
       ter parents. He had been removed from his biological parents'
       custody at an early age because of neglect, and he has been in
       several foster homes. His foster parents report that he is sullen
       and rarely smiles. He often becomes irritable, and they are un-
       able to console him. He appears to interact normally with his
       peers. Which of the following is the most likely diagnosis?

       A. Posttraumatic stress disorder (PTSD).
       B. Autism spectrum disorder.
       C. Reactive attachment disorder.
       D. Adjustment disorder with depressed mood.
       E. Disinhibited social engagement disorder.

9.2    A 6-year-old girl is brought to a child psychiatrist by her new fos-
       ter parents. She had been taken from her biological parents' cus-
       tody at an early age because of neglect, and she has been in
       multiple previous foster homes. Since moving to her new home,
       her foster parents have noticed that she will initiate conversa-
       tions with strangers at the supermarket. She once attempted to
       go home with another family. During the interview, the child
       jumps on the psychiatrist's lap and begins stroking her back.
       Testing has shown that she has a mild intellectual disability, and
       there is no history of a mood disorder. Which of the following is
       the best diagnosis?

       A. PTSD.
       B. Intellectual disability.

C. Bipolar I disorder.

D. Adjustment disorder with depressed mood.

E. Disinhibited social engagement disorder.

9.3 Which of the following is the most common precipitating event for women diagnosed with PTSD?

A. Natural disaster.

B. Experiencing a fire.

C. Physical or sexual assault.

D. Hospitalization in an intensive care unit.

E. Combat.

9.4 Which of the following symptom clusters is *not* required for a PTSD diagnosis?

A. Presence of intrusion symptoms associated with the traumatic event(s).

B. Dissociative reactions such as derealization or depersonalization.

C. Persistent avoidance of stimuli associated with the traumatic event(s).

D. Negative alterations in cognitions and mood.

E. Marked alterations in arousal and reactivity.

9.5 Which of the following is the best medication choice for PTSD?

A. Sertraline.

B. Venlafaxine.

C. Diazepam.

D. Prazosin.

E. Lithium.

9.6 Which of the following statements is true of eye movement desensitization and reprocessing (EMDR) therapy?

A. It is effective for treating adjustment disorders.

B. It is effective in reducing PTSD symptoms by providing patients skills to control anxiety and counter dysfunctional thoughts.

C. Research suggests that its efficacy is driven by exposure carefully integrated with eye movements.

D. Research suggests that its efficacy is driven by the exposure component.

E. Research suggests that its efficacy is driven by the eye movements.

9.7 A 24-year-old man seeks the help of a psychiatrist because of problems with irritability and feeling "on guard" since a motor vehicle accident 2 weeks earlier. Luckily, he sustained only minor physical injuries, but his vehicle was destroyed. Since the accident, he has felt out of sorts and has developed intrusive memories and nightmares about the event. He has been using public transportation to get to work and now avoids going by the scene of the accident. Which of the following is the most likely diagnosis?

A. PTSD.
B. Acute stress disorder.
C. Adjustment disorder with anxious features.
D. Unspecified anxiety disorder.
E. None of the above.

9.8 A 17-year-old boy whose parents divorced 2 months earlier is brought to a therapist by his mother. He has always been a good student, but his grades have dropped, and he has been getting into fights at school over the past month. There is no history of behavioral problems. He says that he isn't depressed, and there have been no changes in his appetite, sleep, or activity level. He answers "I don't know" to most of the therapist's questions. Which of the following is the most likely diagnosis?

A. PTSD.
B. Acute stress disorder.
C. Adjustment disorder.
D. Major depressive disorder.
E. Reactive attachment disorder.

9.9 Which of the following is the most likely stressor for adults with adjustment disorder?

A. Separation or divorce.
B. Motor vehicle accident.
C. Sexual assault.
D. Terrorist attack.
E. Torture.

9.10  Which of the following is required for a diagnosis of adjustment disorder?

A. A stressor.
B. Depressive symptoms.
C. Anxious symptoms.
D. Disturbance of conduct.
E. None of the above.

9.11  Which of the following is the best treatment for an adjustment disorder?

A. Sedative-hypnotics.
B. SSRIs.
C. Second-generation antipsychotics.
D. Supportive psychotherapy.
E. Cognitive-behavioral therapy.

# ——CHAPTER 10——

# Somatic Symptom Disorders and Dissociative Disorders

10.1    A 30-year-old man presents to his primary care physician with a new concern that he could have a brain tumor. He reports that for the past week he has had tingling on his scalp. He had a mild headache the day before that resolved with ibuprofen. At his last visit a few months ago, he was concerned that he had pancreatic cancer because he noticed a small area of yellow discoloration on his upper arm. Which of the following is the most likely diagnosis?

     A. Somatic symptom disorder.
     B. Illness anxiety disorder.
     C. Factitious disorder.
     D. Conversion disorder.
     E. Malingering.

10.2    A 24-year-old woman is referred for a neurology consultation for evaluation of spells that began 2 months earlier. She reports having "seizures" two or three times a week characterized by bilateral arm flapping without impairment of consciousness or loss of bowel or bladder control. The electroencephalogram is negative for epileptiform activity. Routine laboratory studies are unremarkable. Which of the following is the most likely diagnosis?

     A. Somatic symptom disorder.
     B. Convulsive disorder.

C. Factitious disorder.
D. Conversion disorder.
E. Malingering.

10.3 What is the minimum number of symptoms required for a diagnosis of somatic symptom disorder?

A. One.
B. Two.
C. Four.
D. Six.
E. Eight.

10.4 A 60-year-old man receiving disability benefits sees his family physician in follow-up for chronic pain. He reports pain in multiple joints and often requests higher dosages of his opioid pain medication for better pain relief. Diagnostic studies show only changes consistent with normal aging. The patient's primary concern is with pain, and there is no evidence that he misuses his medications. He has been amenable to trying interventions such as physical therapy or cognitive-behavioral therapy, although they have not led to improvement in his pain. Which of the following is the most likely diagnosis?

A. Pain disorder.
B. Somatic symptom disorder.
C. Opioid use disorder.
D. Conversion disorder.
E. Malingering.

10.5 A 19-year-old man presents to his family physician, convinced that his intestines are rotting and that he may already be dead. He is not able to cite any symptoms that give rise to this conviction. Physical examination and routine laboratory tests are normal. The patient does not accept his physician's reassurance that he is healthy. Which of the following is the most likely diagnosis?

A. Somatic symptom disorder.
B. Illness anxiety disorder.
C. Schizophrenia.
D. Malingering.
E. Unspecified somatic symptom disorder.

10.6 A psychiatrist is asked to consult on a 25-year-old man admitted to a neurological service for sudden onset of lower-extremity weakness. The patient reports that he is unable to walk, although diagnostic studies have not shown any physical reason for the symptoms. The patient asks if he will ever get any better. How should the psychiatrist respond?

A. "Your condition will most likely improve with time."
B. "You will most likely be permanently disabled."
C. "Your prognosis is guarded."
D. "It is too early to draw any conclusion."
E. "It will depend on your willingness to engage in cognitive-behavioral therapy."

10.7 A 55-year-old woman sees her family physician for an annual physical examination. During a symptom review, she reports chronic dyspepsia. She had the same complaint during her last three visits. A medical workup for her symptom was negative 3 years ago. She is not preoccupied with this symptom, and her social and occupational functioning is normal. The physician considers diagnosing somatic symptom disorder because there is no obvious medical explanation for her complaint. Her medical student, fresh from a psychiatry clerkship, objects and says that it would be inappropriate. Why so?

A. Patients with somatic symptom disorder must have multiple somatic complaints.
B. The patient's lack of interest in her symptoms makes a conversion disorder more likely.
C. The physician has not investigated possible motivations for secondary gain or to play the patient role.
D. The diagnosis of somatic symptom disorder requires the patient to have significant preoccupation or personal investment in his or her symptoms.
E. The medical student is wrong, and it is appropriate to diagnose this patient with somatic symptom disorder.

10.8 Which of the following is the recommended treatment for somatic symptom disorder?

A. Selective serotonin reuptake inhibitors.
B. Benzodiazepine tranquilizers.

C. Regularly scheduled visits with the same physician.
D. Referral to specialists in order to provide higher levels of care.
E. Aggressive medical workups to offer greater reassurance to patients.

10.9   A psychiatrist is asked to see a 25-year-old man with chronic renal failure admitted to a general medical floor for complications resulting from poor compliance with recommended dialysis. He shows a fair understanding of his medical condition but says that he just feels like taking a day off from dialysis every now and then. Further evaluation shows no evidence of an underlying depression, anxiety disorder, cognitive impairment, psychosis, or personality disorder. Which of the following is the most likely diagnosis?

A. Psychological factors affecting other medical conditions.
B. Factitious disorder.
C. Malingering.
D. Unspecified depressive disorder.
E. Somatic symptom disorder.

10.10  A psychiatrist is asked to see a 25-year-old man with chronic renal failure admitted to a general medical floor for complications resulting from poor compliance with recommended dialysis. He has demanded to leave against medical advice. He has been threatening and verbally abusing staff members. He has fair understanding of his medical condition and is not delirious or confused. Which of the following is the best explanation for his behavior?

A. Psychological factors affecting other medical conditions.
B. Malingering.
C. Unspecified depressive disorder.
D. Somatic symptom disorder.
E. Personal choice in the absence of a mental disorder.

10.11  A 10-year-old boy receives several new video games for his birthday. The following day he tells his mother that he does not feel up to going to school because of stomach upset, although he appears well. His mother gives him a thermometer to check his temperature and leaves the room. When she comes back, the thermometer shows a temperature of 112°F. Which of the following is the most likely diagnosis?

A. Factitious disorder.
B. Malingering.
C. Somatic symptom disorder.
D. Separation anxiety disorder.
E. Psychological factors affecting other medical conditions.

10.12 Which personality disorder is frequently comorbid with dissociative identity disorder?

A. Schizotypal personality disorder.
B. Schizoid personality disorder.
C. Dependent personality disorder.
D. Borderline personality disorder.
E. Narcissistic personality disorder.

10.13 What is the standard treatment for depersonalization/derealization disorder?

A. A benzodiazepine.
B. Fluoxetine.
C. A second-generation antipsychotic.
D. Cognitive-behavioral therapy.
E. There is no standard treatment.

10.14 A 19-year-old college student reports that for the past 2 weeks, since smoking cannabis for the first time, she has felt cut off from herself. She feels that she is watching herself go through the motions and feels unable to connect with her experiences. She did not feel this way before smoking cannabis. Which of the following is the best diagnosis?

A. Dissociative identity disorder.
B. Depersonalization/derealization disorder.
C. Dissociative amnesia.
D. Substance-induced mood disorder.
E. Schizophrenia.

10.15 A 35-year-old man presents to the emergency department. He shows the staff his driver's license and requests help because he has forgotten who he is and where he lives. His driver's license shows that he lives in a town more than 100 miles away. A medical workup including brain imaging is unremarkable. Neuropsychological assessment shows gaps in his ability to recall autobiographical information, but formal testing of memory is normal. Which of the following is the most likely diagnosis?

A. Dissociative identity disorder.
B. Depersonalization/derealization disorder.
C. Dissociative amnesia.
D. Posttraumatic stress disorder.
E. Factitious disorder.

# —CHAPTER 11—

# Feeding and Eating Disorders

11.1  A mother reports to a pediatrician that her 4-year-old son has been eating small quantities of dirt and pebbles from the garden at home. Which of the following is the most likely diagnosis?

A. Pica.
B. Rumination disorder.
C. Avoidant/restrictive food intake disorder.
D. Other specified feeding disorder.
E. None of the above.

11.2  A mother reports to a pediatrician that her 15-month-old daughter mouths on a variety of inanimate objects in the home. Which of the following is the most likely diagnosis?

A. Pica.
B. Rumination disorder.
C. Avoidant/restrictive food intake disorder.
D. Other specified feeding disorder.
E. None of the above.

11.3  A 7-year-old girl is brought to a pediatric gastroenterologist by her parents. They are concerned because they have noticed that she has been regurgitating swallowed food and then swallowing it again or sometimes expelling it. The girl does not report symptoms such as heartburn or stomach pain. Her food intake is appropriate for her age, and she does not appear preoccupied with her body shape or size. A medical workup is unremarkable. Which of the following is the most likely diagnosis?

A. Pica.
B. Rumination disorder.
C. Avoidant/restrictive food intake disorder.
D. Bulimia nervosa.
E. Anorexia nervosa.

11.4 An 11-year-old boy with autism spectrum disorder is brought to a pediatrician because his mother is concerned about his poor appetite. He has always been a picky eater, but his mother is especially concerned because it's about time for his "growth spurt." The boy is thin but not emaciated and is of normal height. He tells his doctor that he's not very interested in food and that he finds the textures of most foods unappetizing. He denies being preoccupied with being thin, and there is no evidence of depression. Which of the following is the most likely diagnosis?

A. Pica.
B. Rumination disorder.
C. Avoidant/restrictive food intake disorder.
D. Bulimia nervosa.
E. Anorexia nervosa.

11.5 A 50-year-old man is brought to his family physician at his wife's insistence. She is concerned that he has lost 15 pounds in the past month and stopped going to work. He "barely eats a thing," she says. The man reports that he no longer has any interest in anything. He spends most of the day watching TV but does not pay much attention to the shows. He complains of poor sleep, waking up at about 3:00 A.M. every morning and not being able to go back to sleep. He displays a restricted affect. Which of the following is the most likely diagnosis?

A. Pica.
B. Rumination disorder.
C. Avoidant/restrictive food intake disorder.
D. Major depressive disorder.
E. Anorexia nervosa.

11.6 What is the key difference between anorexia nervosa and bulimia nervosa?

A. Presence of bingeing behavior.
B. Presence of purging behavior.
C. Preoccupation with one's body weight.
D. Current body weight.
E. Personality traits.

11.7 Which of the following physical examination findings is *not* typical of anorexia nervosa?

A. Tachycardia.
B. Hypokalemia.
C. Amenorrhea.
D. Hair loss.
E. Constipation.

11.8 Which brain region plays an important role in regulating feeding behavior?

A. Thalamus.
B. Hypothalamus.
C. Pineal gland.
D. Amygdala.
E. Entorhinal cortex.

11.9 Which of the following physical examination findings would suggest a diagnosis of bulimia nervosa or the binge-eating/purging subtype of anorexia nervosa rather than another eating disorder?

A. Constipation.
B. Decreased thyroid-stimulating hormone.
C. Dental caries.
D. Amenorrhea.
E. Hair loss.

11.10 During a routine health maintenance examination, a 30-year-old man tells his family physician that he has been having trouble losing weight. He reports that three to four times each week, he loses control of his eating and consumes a large quantity of food such that he feels physically uncomfortable afterward. He is overweight and has some concern about his body image, but he denies being obsessed with being thin. He denies excessive exercise or other compensatory behaviors. Which of the following is the most likely diagnosis?

A. Binge-eating disorder.
B. Rumination disorder.
C. Avoidant/restrictive food intake disorder.
D. Bulimia nervosa.
E. Anorexia nervosa.

11.11  Which antidepressant is contraindicated in patients with eating disorders?

A. Fluoxetine.
B. Sertraline.
C. Bupropion.
D. Venlafaxine.
E. Mirtazapine.

11.12  Which medication is U.S. Food and Drug Administration (FDA) approved for the treatment of bulimia nervosa?

A. Sertraline.
B. Fluoxetine.
C. Lithium.
D. Venlafaxine.
E. Olanzapine.

11.13  What is the first objective in treating an eating disorder?

A. Correct faulty cognitions about body image.
B. Modify distorted eating behaviors.
C. Restore nutritional status.
D. Correct unhealthy home environment that gives rise to the disorder.
E. Initiate SSRI to address disturbed serotonergic neurotransmission.

# — CHAPTER 12 —

# Sleep-Wake Disorders

12.1   Which sleep stage is characterized by rapid conjugate eye movements, reduced muscle tone, and respiratory and cardiac rate fluctuations with loss of body temperature control?

A. Stage N1 (non–rapid eye movement [NREM] 1).
B. Stage N2 (NREM 2).
C. Stage N3 (NREM 3).
D. Stage R (REM).
E. All the above.

12.2   Which procedure can be used to measure excessive daytime sleepiness?

A. Polysomnography.
B. Multiple Sleep Latency Test.
C. Electroencephalogram (EEG).
D. A sleep log.
E. Neuropsychological evaluation.

12.3   As part of a cognitive-behavioral approach to treating insomnia, which of the following is *not* a standard recommendation?

A. Discontinuing the intake of alcohol, caffeine, and sedative-hypnotics.
B. Avoiding reading, working, or watching TV in bed.
C. Staying awake in bed for long periods of time until sleep onset occurs.
D. Going to bed and waking up at the same time every day, even on weekends.
E. Avoiding napping.

12.4    What is the treatment of choice for insomnia disorder?

   A. Temazepam.
   B. Trazodone.
   C. Diphenhydramine.
   D. Zolpidem.
   E. Cognitive-behavioral therapy for insomnia (CBTi).

12.5    A 35-year-old man complains to his family physician of difficulty falling asleep for the past 8 months. It takes him up to an hour to fall asleep, and he reports feeling fatigued throughout the day. He sometimes feels irritable but denies significant depression. He does not snore, nor does he feel sleepy during the day. He stopped his caffeine intake a couple of months ago after reading about sleep hygiene on the Internet. Which of the following is the most likely diagnosis?

   A. Hypersomnolence disorder.
   B. Narcolepsy.
   C. Insomnia disorder.
   D. Obstructive sleep apnea.
   E. Other specified insomnia disorder.

12.6    Which of the following suggests hypersomnolence disorder rather than narcolepsy?

   A. Daytime napping.
   B. Decreased REM sleep latency.
   C. Spells of brief loss of muscle tone (hypotonia).
   D. Hypocretin deficiency.
   E. Sleep drunkenness.

12.7    A 22-year-old woman presents to a sleep disorders clinic. She reports that she is groggy most every morning, and it takes her more than an hour to become alert. She sleeps 9–10 hours at night. She feels sleepy during the day and will sometimes take a 1- to 2-hour nap. She denies episodes of cataplexy or excessive caffeine use. Which treatment may be effective for this patient?

   A. Selective serotonin reuptake inhibitor (SSRI).
   B. Benzodiazepine.
   C. Stimulant.

D. Nonbenzodiazepine hypnotic.

E. Antihistamine.

12.8 What causes narcolepsy?

A. Loss of cholinergic cells in the nucleus basalis.

B. Loss of hypocretin-secreting cells in the hypothalamus.

C. Decrease in REM sleep latency.

D. Poor sleep hygiene.

E. The cause is unknown.

12.9 Which of the following is an effective treatment for sleep attacks associated with narcolepsy?

A. Tricyclic antidepressant.

B. Sodium oxybate.

C. Methylphenidate.

D. Zolpidem.

E. Improved sleep hygiene.

12.10 What is the technical term used for a decrease in airflow during sleeping?

A. Apnea.

B. Hypopnea.

C. Cheyne-Stokes breathing.

D. Hyperventilation.

E. None of the above.

12.11 A 45-year-old obese man complains to his family physician of chronic trouble with sleep maintenance. He falls asleep easily at night but awakens 10–20 times throughout the night. He feels fatigued during the day and occasionally takes short naps. He says that his wife tells him that he snores loudly at times but not on most nights. He sleeps in a quiet dark room and goes to bed at about the same time on most nights but might stay up 30–45 minutes later than usual on weekends. His blood pressure is normal. He drinks two to three cups of coffee in the morning and may have a 12 oz can of soda in the late afternoon. What is the best next step in management of this patient?

A. Prescribe a benzodiazepine.

B. Have the patient eliminate caffeine intake.

C. Order a Multiple Sleep Latency Test.

D. Order a polysomnogram.

E. Counsel the patient on sleep hygiene and follow up in 3 months.

12.12 Which of the following is *not* suggestive of obstructive sleep apnea hypopnea?

A. Snoring.

B. Daytime fatigue.

C. Apneic episodes.

D. Crescendo-decrescendo variation in tidal volume.

E. Difficult-to-control hypertension.

12.13 Which of the following treatment methods can be used for refractory cases of obstructive sleep apnea hypopnea?

A. Weight-loss counseling.

B. CPAP.

C. Sedative-hypnotics.

D. Respiratory assist devices.

E. Hypoglossal nerve stimulator.

12.14 A 50-year-old woman who has chronic obstructive pulmonary disease reports to her family physician that she has morning headache and daytime fatigue. Routine laboratory studies are remarkable for elevated carbon dioxide ($CO_2$). A polysomnogram shows periods of decreased respiration. Which of the following is the most likely diagnosis?

A. Obstructive sleep apnea hypopnea.

B. Central sleep apnea.

C. Sleep-related hypoventilation.

D. Hypersomnolence disorder.

E. Narcolepsy.

12.15 A 27-year-old man who works nights at a convenience store reports to his family physician that his energy is chronically low and he has little motivation. He can only sleep 4–6 hours during the day. He tries to maintain a diurnal schedule on his days off on the weekend but has trouble falling asleep at night. Which of the following is the most likely diagnosis?

A. Insomnia disorder.

B. Obstructive sleep apnea hypopnea.

C. Hypersomnolence disorder.
D. Circadian rhythm sleep-wake disorder.
E. Narcolepsy.

12.16 What is the best treatment for circadian rhythm sleep-wake disorder, shift work type?

A. Improved sleep hygiene.
B. Methylphenidate to improve alertness.
C. Zolpidem to assist with daytime sleep.
D. Melatonin to regulate circadian rhythm.
E. Discontinue shift work.

12.17 What is the DSM-5 diagnosis used for both sleepwalking and sleep terrors?

A. NREM sleep arousal disorder.
B. REM sleep behavior disorder.
C. Parasomnia.
D. Circadian rhythm sleep-wake disorder.
E. None of the above.

12.18 A 15-year-old boy has recurrent vivid dreams with frightening violent content. He wakes up in the morning with a racing heart and heavy breathing, but he does not scream or act out. Which of the following is the most likely diagnosis?

A. REM sleep behavior disorder.
B. NREM sleep arousal disorder, sleep terror type.
C. Nightmare disorder.
D. Parasomnia.
E. None of the above.

12.19 Which sleep disorder is associated with Parkinson's disease, Lewy body dementia, and multiple system atrophy?

A. REM sleep behavior disorder.
B. NREM sleep arousal disorder, sleep terror type.
C. Nightmare disorder.
D. Parasomnia.
E. Central sleep apnea.

12.20 A 31-year-old woman reports to her family physician that she has the uncomfortable sensation of having to move her legs at night when she is in bed. She says that she does not sleep well because of this. She wonders if something can be given to treat her condition. Which of the following can be used to treat this condition?

A. Zolpidem.
B. Pramipexole.
C. Sodium oxybate.
D. Clonazepam.
E. Imipramine.

# —CHAPTER 13—

# Sexual Dysfunction, Gender Dysphoria, and Paraphilic Disorders

13.1 How long should a disorder of sexual function be present prior to diagnosis?

    A. At least 18 months.
    B. At least 4 months.
    C. At least 1 month.
    D. At least 6 months.
    E. At least 1 year.

13.2 Which of the following would preclude a diagnosis of a sexual dysfunction?

    A. Severe relationship stress.
    B. A nonsexual mental disorder that would account for symptoms.
    C. Disturbance caused by substance use or medication.
    D. Disturbance caused by medical condition such as diabetes.
    E. Any of the above.

13.3 A 22-year-old man reports to his family physician that he has had persistent difficulty achieving orgasm during intercourse with his partner. He has no trouble attaining an erection. The problem has been ongoing since the relationship began about a year ago. He does not have any difficulty achieving orgasm during mas-

turbation and reports that otherwise his relationship is going
well. He does not take any medications. Which of the following
is the most likely diagnosis?

A. No diagnosis.
B. Other specified sexual dysfunction.
C. Delayed ejaculation.
D. Male hypoactive sexual desire disorder.
E. Erectile disorder.

13.4    A 28-year-old man reports to his family physician that he has had
persistent difficulty achieving orgasm both with his partner and
while masturbating. He has no trouble attaining an erection. His
problem has been ongoing since the relationship began about a
year ago. He reports that otherwise his relationship is going well.
He takes fluoxetine but no other medication. Which of the following is the most likely diagnosis?

A. Medication-induced sexual dysfunction.
B. Other specified sexual dysfunction.
C. Delayed ejaculation.
D. Male hypoactive sexual desire disorder.
E. Erectile disorder.

13.5    A 30-year-old woman reports to her family physician of ongoing
sexual difficulties with her partner for the last several years. She
experiences vaginal and pelvic pain during intercourse. She denies that there is difficulty achieving vaginal penetration, and she
is not sure about tightening of her pelvic muscles during penetration. Which of the following is the most likely diagnosis?

A. Dyspareunia.
B. Vaginismus.
C. Genito-pelvic pain disorder.
D. Female sexual interest/arousal disorder.
E. None of the above.

13.6    A 50-year-old man reports to his family physician that in the past
few months he has had a new onset of erectile dysfunction during intercourse and masturbation. He is baffled about why it is
happening at his age and reports that his sexual interest remains
strong. He has been feeling more jittery than usual over the past

few months, and he reports occasional palpitations and diaphoresis on review of systems. What is the next best step in management of this patient?

A. Refer to a psychiatrist.
B. Start an SSRI.
C. Refer to a psychotherapist.
D. Order thyroid-stimulating hormone test.
E. None of the above.

13.7 What medication can be used to treat premature ejaculation?

A. Sildenafil.
B. Alprostadil.
C. Vardenafil.
D. Paroxetine.
E. Tadalafil.

13.8 Which of the following medications is a standard treatment for erectile disorder?

A. Vardenafil.
B. Paroxetine.
C. Dibucaine.
D. Testosterone.
E. Topical estrogen.

13.9 Which of the following is *not* typical of gender dysphoria?

A. Onset occurs in childhood.
B. The child prefers to play with children of the same gender.
C. The child expresses a strong desire to be rid of one's primary and secondary sexual characteristics because of incongruence between one's expressed and experienced gender.
D. The child expresses strong preference for cross-sex roles in make-believe play.
E. The child shows a strong preference for games, toys, and activities stereotypically associated with the opposite gender.

13.10 A 40-year-old man reports to his psychiatrist that he enjoys dressing in women's clothing prior to intercourse, but this has caused conflict with his wife. He identifies himself as heterosexual, and he reports that he is comfortable being male. Which of the following is the most likely diagnosis?

A. Gender dysphoria.
B. Transvestic disorder.
C. Voyeuristic disorder.
D. Exhibitionistic disorder.
E. Frotteuristic disorder.

13.11  What is the DSM-5 term for an anomalous sexual activity preference?

A. Paraphilic disorder.
B. Paraphilia.
C. Infantilism.
D. Infantilism disorder.
E. None of the above.

13.12  Which of the following has *not* been used in the treatment of paraphilic disorders?

A. Masturbatory satiation.
B. SSRIs.
C. Behavioral activation.
D. Cognitive-behavioral therapy.
E. Couples therapy.

# — CHAPTER 14 —

# Disruptive, Impulse-Control, and Conduct Disorders

14.1 A 7-year-old girl is brought to a therapist by her mother. Her mother says the girl is always touchy and irritable and gets very angry when told to do anything. The behavior has been present for more than a year. When asked about her symptoms, the girl says that it's her mother's fault for always making her mad. She has not engaged in any stealing, fire setting, or runaway behavior. She gets along with her peers, and her grades in school are good. Which of the following is the most likely diagnosis?

   A. Antisocial personality disorder.
   B. Conduct disorder.
   C. Attention-deficit/hyperactivity disorder (ADHD).
   D. Oppositional defiant disorder.
   E. Normal development.

14.2 A 16-year-old boy with an autism spectrum disorder is brought to the emergency department by his family. His father reports that he broke two windows and smashed several plates in the kitchen after his father told him that he would not be able to use the computer for the next day because he had failed to clean up his room. The boy has had similar destructive outbursts when his computer privileges have been restricted in the past. Ordinarily, he is quiet, keeps to himself, and does not bother others. He does not have a history of truancy, fire setting, cruelty to animals, or fighting. Which of the following is the most likely diagnosis?

A. Oppositional defiant disorder.
B. Conduct disorder.
C. Antisocial personality disorder.
D. Intermittent explosive disorder.
E. No additional diagnosis apart from autism spectrum disorder.

14.3  A 16-year-old boy is brought to a psychiatrist at his parents' insistence for problem behavior ongoing for 3 years. He has had repeated legal trouble for acts of vandalism, and he has been expelled from school several times for fighting. He is failing all his classes. He tells the psychiatrist that he doesn't care about his schoolwork and has no remorse for his actions. What DSM-5 specifier is appropriate for this form of conduct disorder?

A. With limited prosocial emotions.
B. With antisocial personality features.
C. With psychopathic personality features.
D. Childhood-onset type.
E. DSM-5 does not have a descriptor for such cases.

14.4  A 35-year-old man is charged with arson after burning down a building he owned in order to collect insurance money. He has no previous criminal history, and his work history has been stable. He denies any previous episodes of fire setting. Which of the following options best explains his behavior?

A. Antisocial personality disorder.
B. There is no psychiatric diagnosis.
C. Pyromania.
D. Intermittent explosive disorder.
E. Conduct disorder.

14.5  What is the treatment for pyromania?

A. Cognitive-behavioral therapy.
B. Selective serotonin reuptake inhibitor (SSRI).
C. Mood stabilizer such as carbamazepine.
D. Second-generation antipsychotic such as risperidone.
E. There is no standard treatment for pyromania.

14.6 A 24-year-old woman comes forward to establish care with a therapist. She reports a problem with compulsive stealing. She has taken small items of modest value from stores and from the homes of friends and family on many occasions since adolescence. She reports feeling tension before the theft and a sense of gratification afterward. She is motivated to change her behavior because she was recently given probation for shoplifting. She denies any other criminal activity or interpersonal problems. Which of the following is the most likely diagnosis?

A. Conduct disorder.
B. Antisocial personality disorder.
C. Kleptomania.
D. Compulsive shopping.
E. Oppositional defiant disorder.

14.7 All but which of the following might be beneficial for patients with intermittent explosive disorder?

A. Fluoxetine.
B. Oxcarbazepine.
C. Cognitive-behavioral therapy.
D. Benzodiazepine tranquilizers.
E. Fluoxetine and oxcarbazepine.

14.8 Naltrexone has shown to be more effective than placebo for treating which of the following?

A. Intermittent explosive disorder.
B. Conduct disorder.
C. Kleptomania.
D. Pyromania.
E. Oppositional defiant disorder.

# —CHAPTER 15—

# Substance-Related and Addictive Disorders

15.1 A 48-year-old woman reports to her family physician that she has been drinking a bottle of wine two to three times per week for the past 3 years. She has not been successful in her attempts to cut back her drinking, and her drinking has led to conflicts with her family. She is occasionally late for work when she is hungover but has never had symptoms of alcohol withdrawal. Which of the following is the best diagnosis?

A. Alcohol use disorder.
B. Alcohol dependence.
C. Alcohol abuse.
D. Alcoholism.
E. Alcohol abuse disorder.

15.2 Which neurotransmitter plays a key role in the development of all substance use disorders?

A. Serotonin.
B. Acetylcholine.
C. β-Endorphin.
D. Norepinephrine.
E. Dopamine.

15.3 Which neurotransmitter plays a role specifically in the development of opioid use disorders?

A. Dopamine.
B. β-Endorphin.
C. Acetylcholine.
D. Serotonin.
E. Norepinephrine.

15.4 A 17-year-old girl is referred for treatment of an alcohol use disorder. She drinks nearly every day (mostly beer and wine) and drinks to intoxication twice weekly. Her father drinks excessively, and the family receives government assistance. One reason she gives for her drinking is that her friends also drink, and it is hard for her not to go along with them. Which of the following variables is associated with a lesser risk for developing an alcohol use disorder?

A. Low socioeconomic status.
B. Susceptibility to peer influence.
C. Female sex.
D. Younger age.
E. Parental alcoholism.

15.5 How many positive responses on a CAGE test are needed to indicate that a person might have an alcohol use disorder?

A. One.
B. Two.
C. Three.
D. Four.
E. The CAGE test is not a good screening test for alcohol use disorders.

15.6 Which of the following develops as a late-stage consequence of an alcohol use disorder?

A. Decreased work productivity.
B. Moodiness or irritability.
C. Palmar erythema.
D. Rosacea.
E. Jaundice.

15.7 A 45-year-old man reports a 10-year history of heavy alcohol consumption to his family physician. He tells his physician that he is not as "sharp" as he used to be before he started drinking and that he has some mild difficulties with everyday memory tasks. He asks his doctor if these memory problems will be permanent. What is the best response?

A. "Even if you stop drinking, these memory problems are likely to be irreversible but not progressive."
B. "Even if you stop drinking, these memory problems are likely to be irreversible and progressive."
C. "If you stop drinking now, these memory problems may partially reverse."
D. "If you stop drinking now, your memory will likely fully recover."
E. None of the above.

15.8 What percentage of motor vehicle deaths are related to alcohol use?

A. 10%.
B. 20%.
C. 30%.
D. 40%.
E. >50%.

15.9 Which of the following are the last symptoms to develop during the course of severe alcohol withdrawal?

A. Delirium, fever, autonomic hyperarousal.
B. Auditory, visual, tactile hallucinations in the presence of a clear sensorium.
C. Seizures.
D. Anxiety, tremor, nausea.
E. Increased heart rate and blood pressure.

15.10 A psychiatrist is called to evaluate a 38-year-old man for admission to a psychiatric unit for alcohol detoxification and treatment of depression. He has been drinking large quantities of vodka daily for several months. He previously drank three to four beers nearly daily for almost 5 years. His last drink was 6 hours ago. He is currently pleasant and cooperative. He is fully oriented and in no distress. The psychiatrist asks the man if he has ever had delirium tremens (DTs). He responds, "Oh yeah, I've got the shakes right now," and he holds out his hands to show the psychiatrist his mild tremor. How shall the psychiatrist proceed?

A. Recommend admission to intensive care because DTs can be fatal.
B. Admit the patient to psychiatry for alcohol rehabilitation.
C. Administer chlordiazepoxide now.
D. Collect additional information such as if the man has ever had confusion and fever during withdrawal or had become agitated.
E. None of the above.

15.11 Which medication used to treat alcohol dependence works by inhibiting aldehyde dehydrogenase?

A. Naltrexone.
B. Disulfiram.
C. Acamprosate.
D. Chlordiazepoxide.
E. Lorazepam.

15.12 A 20-year-old student sees his internist for anxiety symptoms. He reports that he has started worrying about everything since he started college about 2 years ago. He has trouble falling asleep and staying asleep nearly every night. His mood is mildly irritable, and he appears restless. He does not smoke, use alcohol, or use illicit drugs. He reports that he drinks eight or more cups of coffee daily to help him stay motivated when studying, with his last cup around 8:00–10:00 P.M. Which of the following is the most likely diagnosis?

A. Generalized anxiety disorder.
B. Bipolar I disorder.
C. Caffeine-induced anxiety disorder.
D. Panic disorder.
E. Insomnia disorder.

15.13 Which of the following is *not* associated with cannabis use?

A. Increased risk of developing schizophrenia.
B. Increased risk of smoking cigarettes and abusing other drugs.

C. Tachycardia, dry mouth, and conjunctivitis during intoxication.

D. Flashbacks between periods of use.

E. Feeling that time has slowed and increased appetite during intoxication.

15.14 A 19-year-old man presents to the emergency department complaining of acute-onset severe anxiety, confusion, time expansion, and vivid visual hallucinations. He took LSD for the first time 3 hours ago and is very uncomfortable, but he is cooperative in interview. His pupils are dilated, and he has mild tachycardia. Reassurance fails to calm him down. Which of the following is the next best step in managing this case?

A. Give an antipsychotic.

B. Give a benzodiazepine.

C. Give clonidine.

D. Give naltrexone.

E. Refer the man to a substance use treatment program.

15.15 A 30-year-old man requests help for an opioid abuse disorder. He has used large quantities of prescription narcotics obtained on the streets and will also inject heroin when it is available. He has tried to quit these drugs on his own several times without success. Which of the following is the best option to treat his opioid use disorder and reduce his risk of relapse and criminal activity?

A. Referral to Narcotics Anonymous.

B. Detoxification with clonidine followed by outpatient counseling.

C. Referral to a methadone or buprenorphine maintenance program following detoxification.

D. Prescribing naltrexone.

E. Detoxification with clonidine followed by referral to an intensive outpatient program.

15.16 A 26-year-old woman comes to your office seeking help for anxiety and panic attacks. She was last seen by your colleague a week ago, but she reports that she has lost her prescription for alprazolam. She asks you to write a new prescription for alprazolam 3 mg four times daily. She reports that nothing else works and that she has allergies to the selective serotonin reuptake inhibitors. Which of the following is *not* a valid reason to have serious concerns about prescribing alprazolam to this patient?

A. Concern about doctor-shopping behavior.
B. Report that "nothing else works."
C. Report of severe allergies to other medications commonly used to treat anxiety.
D. Report of a lost prescription.
E. Lethality of benzodiazepines in overdose.

15.17 A 23-year-old man with no psychiatric history is brought to the emergency department by the police for agitated and disorganized behavior. He is paranoid and believes that the government is sending him messages through a microchip that was implanted in one of his teeth. He has not slept for 3 days. He is distractible in interview but otherwise oriented. A urine drug screen is positive for amphetamine. He is otherwise medically stable and is admitted to the psychiatry unit. What is the best course of treatment for this patient's psychotic symptoms?

A. Supportive care and possibly short-term use of antipsychotic.
B. Antipsychotic therapy for 6 months.
C. Cognitive-behavioral psychotherapy.
D. Imipramine.
E. Lithium.

15.18 Your patient tells you that he plans to stop smoking cigarettes because he realizes that it constitutes a major health hazard. He asks for your advice about how to quit successfully. Which of the following is most likely to help your patient quit smoking?

A. Bupropion.
B. Quitting "cold turkey."
C. Nicotine gum.
D. Varenicline.
E. A combination of nicotine gum and varenicline.

15.19 What form of therapy for substance use disorders rewards patients for appropriate behavior (e.g., giving patients who submit clean urine samples vouchers that can be exchanged for retail goods and services)?

A. Contingency management.
B. Motivational interviewing.
C. Cognitive-behavioral therapy.
D. Behavioral activation.
E. Twelve-step program.

15.20 Which of the following treatments has a role in treating gambling disorder?

A. Gamblers Anonymous.
B. Naltrexone.
C. Motivational interviewing.
D. Cognitive-behavioral therapy.
E. All the above.

# — CHAPTER 16 —

# Neurocognitive Disorders

16.1    Which of the following is a neurocognitive disorder new to DSM-5?

    A. Social cognitive disorder.

    B. Alzheimer's dementia.

    C. Major cognitive impairment disorder.

    D. Mild neurocognitive disorder.

    E. Dementia disorder.

16.2    Processing speed is a part of which cognitive domain?

    A. Social cognition.

    B. Complex attention.

    C. Learning and memory.

    D. Executive function.

    E. Language.

16.3    Which of the following is *not* a risk factor for delirium?

    A. Use of narcotics.

    B. Recent surgery.

    C. Older age.

    D. Preexisting depression.

    E. Systemic infection.

16.4 Which of the following is *least* consistent with delirium?

A. Fluctuation in mental status throughout the day.
B. Disturbance of memory.
C. Occurrence in a hospitalized patient receiving narcotics.
D. Patient reports of visual and tactile hallucinations.
E. Insidious onset.

16.5 In which of the following patients are benzodiazepines *least* likely to worsen his or her delirium?

A. A highly agitated 25-year-old man hospitalized for 2 weeks for encephalopathy.
B. A calm 32-year-old woman hospitalized for 1 week for pneumonia.
C. A 65-year-old man with a severe alcohol use disorder hospitalized for the past 3 days recovering from abdominal surgery.
D. An agitated 75-year-old woman with sepsis who reports vivid visual hallucinations.
E. Any patient with delirium.

16.6 Which of the following distinguishes a major and mild neurocognitive disorder?

A. Decline in memory from baseline.
B. Presence of attentional difficulties.
C. Presence of impairment on neuropsychological assessment.
D. Acute onset over days.
E. Impairment in ability to live independently.

16.7 What percentage of patients with a major neurocognitive disorder due to Alzheimer's disease develop psychotic symptoms such as hallucinations and delusions as their illness progresses?

A. 1%.
B. 5%.
C. 10%.
D. 25%.
E. 50%.

16.8 A 67-year-old retired accountant presents to his family physician accompanied by his wife. His wife reports that he has been having progressive difficulty remembering appointments and important dates over the past 2 years, and she no longer allows him to drive. There are no current safety concerns at home. Brief cognitive assessment shows that he has impaired short-term recall and difficulty drawing a clock. What is the next best step in management of this case?

A. Referral to a skilled nursing facility.
B. Medical workup.
C. Neuropsychological assessment.
D. Start donepezil.
E. Referral to a psychiatrist to confirm diagnosis of a neurocognitive disorder.

16.9 Which test can distinguish major neurocognitive disorder due to Alzheimer's disease from other neurocognitive disorders?

A. Magnetic resonance imaging (MRI).
B. Functional MRI.
C. Fluorodeoxyglucose positron emission tomography (PET).
D. Lumbar puncture.
E. Alzheimer's disease can only be confirmed on autopsy.

16.10 A 59-year-old woman is brought to her family physician accompanied by her spouse. She has had worsening of short-term memory and progressive apathy over the past month. She also reports low mood, insomnia, and low appetite, and she has lost 10 pounds since the symptoms began. She answers "I don't know" to many basic questions on a brief cognitive assessment. Which of the following medications would be of most benefit to this patient?

A. Donepezil.
B. Tacrine.
C. Sertraline.
D. Aripiprazole.
E. Memantine.

16.11 Which of the following is most specific for Alzheimer's disease?

A. Neurofibrillary tangles.
B. β-Amyloid plaques.
C. Hyperphosphorylated tau protein.
D. Apolipoprotein E polymorphism.
E. All the above are equally specific changes.

16.12 Primary progressive aphasia and a behavioral-variant subtype occur in which neurocognitive disorder?

A. Alzheimer's disease.
B. Frontotemporal neurocognitive disorder.
C. Neurocognitive disorder with Lewy bodies.
D. Vascular neurocognitive disorder.
E. None of the above.

16.13 Which neurocognitive disorder is sometimes associated with rapid eye movement (REM) sleep behavior disorder?

A. Alzheimer's disease.
B. Frontotemporal neurocognitive disorder.
C. Neurocognitive disorder with Lewy bodies.
D. Vascular neurocognitive disorder.
E. None of the above.

16.14 A 67-year-old man is brought in by his family to see his family physician. They are concerned because he has had progressive difficulty keeping up with daily chores at home and is more irritable than usual. He tells the physician that he wouldn't be so irritable if his wife hadn't moved so many of her friends into the house. His wife reports that they live alone, and he seems to see people who aren't there. The patient is oriented and attends to the interview without difficulty. The physician notices that the patient has a shuffling gait. Which of the following is the most likely diagnosis?

A. Alzheimer's disease.
B. Frontotemporal neurocognitive disorder.
C. Neurocognitive disorder with Lewy bodies.
D. Vascular neurocognitive disorder.
E. Dementia.

16.15  A rapid, progressive stepwise cognitive decline suggests which neurocognitive disorder?

A. Alzheimer's disease.
B. Frontotemporal neurocognitive disorder.
C. Neurocognitive disorder with Lewy bodies.
D. Vascular neurocognitive disorder.
E. Delirium.

16.16  A 25-year-old man recently diagnosed with an HIV infection sees his internist to address some concerns. He has read about "HIV dementia," and he asks his physician about his risk of developing this complication. What is the most accurate response?

A. "It's a rare complication, so your risk is low."
B. "You have a high risk of developing this condition at some point."
C. "We can't determine this at the present."
D. "There's a fair chance you may eventually develop some mild cognitive problems, but your risk of developing severe cognitive problems is low."
E. None of the above.

16.17  Which of the following findings is characteristic of Creutzfeldt-Jakob disease?

A. Triphasic complexes on EEG.
B. Diffuse slowing on EEG.
C. Hypocretin deficiency.
D. Degeneration of the mamillary bodies.
E. Hypometabolism of parietal and temporal areas on PET scan.

16.18  Dementia, gait disturbance, and urinary incontinence are the classic triad of which medical condition that can cause a neurocognitive disorder?

A. Pellagra.
B. Prion disease.
C. Subdural hematoma.
D. Alcohol use.
E. Normal-pressure hydrocephalus.

16.19 Which of the following medications is an appropriate choice to help with nighttime agitation, or "sundowning," in patients with neurocognitive disorders?

A. Lithium.
B. Carbamazepine.
C. Divalproex.
D. Trazodone.
E. Chlorpromazine.

16.20 Which of the following cognitive-enhancing drugs works on *N*-methyl-D-aspartate (NMDA) receptors?

A. Donepezil.
B. Tacrine.
C. Memantine.
D. Rivastigmine.
E. Galantamine.

16.21 Why has the U.S. Food and Drug Administration (FDA) issued a black box warning about the use of second-generation antipsychotics in elderly patients with neurocognitive disorders?

A. They are associated with an increased rate of cognitive decline.
B. They are associated with severe gastrointestinal side effects.
C. They are associated with an increased risk of mortality.
D. Liver enzymes must be monitored regularly.
E. They have no benefit for managing disruptive behaviors in patients with neurocognitive disorders.

# ―― CHAPTER 17 ――

# Personality Disorders

17.1  Which was the first DSM to include disturbances of personality?

A. DSM-I.
B. DSM-II.
C. DSM-III.
D. DSM-IV.
E. DSM-5.

17.2  Which of the following is *not* true of the general criteria of a personality disorder?

A. The behavior is consistent with the individual's cultural expectations.
B. It is stable over time with onset in adolescence or early adulthood.
C. The disorder leads to distress or impairment.
D. The disorder is not limited to episodes of illness.
E. All the above are part of the general criteria of a personality disorder.

17.3  A patient has long-standing discrete episodes of mania and depression dating to late adolescence. During manic episodes, he displays elevated mood, decreased sleep, pressured speech, and flight of ideas. The episodes typically result in psychiatric hospitalization. During the manic episodes, he engages in antisocial behavior, including committing assaults and writing bad checks. He is a quiet, law-abiding citizen between episodes of mania. Which of the following is the most likely diagnosis?

A. Antisocial personality disorder.
B. Bipolar I disorder.

C. Personality disorder due to bipolar I disorder.

D. Bipolar I disorder plus antisocial personality disorder.

E. None of the above.

17.4 A patient has long-standing discrete episodes of mania and depression dating back to late adolescence. During the manic episodes, he has elevated mood, decreased sleep, pressured speech, and flight of ideas that typically result in psychiatric hospitalization. He gets into more legal trouble than usual during these periods, but even during periods of euthymia, he tends to engage in illegal activities such as shoplifting and burglary. He has done so since early adolescence, and he does not show any remorse for these actions. Which of the following is the most likely diagnosis?

A. Antisocial personality disorder.

B. Bipolar I disorder.

C. Personality disorder due to bipolar I disorder.

D. Bipolar I disorder plus antisocial personality disorder.

E. None of the above.

17.5 Which of the following personality disorders is *not* a Cluster C personality disorder?

A. Avoidant personality disorder.

B. Obsessive-compulsive personality disorder.

C. Histrionic personality disorder.

D. Dependent personality disorder.

E. All the above are Cluster C personality disorders.

17.6 Which of the following does *not* represent a major personality trait according to personality theorists who favor a dimensional perspective?

A. Extraversion.

B. Agreeableness.

C. Openness to experience.

D. Genuineness.

E. Neuroticism.

17.7 Which of the following personality disorders occurs about equally in men and women?

A. Antisocial personality disorder.
B. Borderline personality disorder.
C. Histrionic personality disorder.
D. Dependent personality disorder.
E. Schizotypal personality disorder.

17.8 Which of the following is the only personality disorder with an age requirement and a requirement that certain childhood behaviors have continuity with adult traits?

A. Antisocial personality disorder.
B. Borderline personality disorder.
C. Avoidant personality disorder.
D. Dependent personality disorder.
E. Schizotypal personality disorder.

17.9 Does the diagnosis of a personality disorder tend to be stable over time?

A. Most personality disorders are diagnostically stable throughout life, but the severity may diminish with age.
B. Most personality disorders are diagnostically stable, and symptom severity is stable.
C. Severity of personality disorders diminishes, and many people will make a full psychosocial recovery.
D. Severity of personality disorders diminishes, but many people will still have some degree of interpersonal dysfunction.
E. None of the above.

17.10 Which of the following has *not* been shown to contribute to the risk of developing a personality disorder?

A. Being a victim of child abuse.
B. Witnessing domestic violence in the home.
C. Parental divorce or separation.
D. Parental absence.
E. Arrested psychosexual development.

17.11 Which of the following personality disorders is associated with impaired smooth pursuit eye movement, impaired performance on tests of executive function, and increased ventricular-brain ratio on computed tomography?

A. Antisocial personality disorder.
B. Borderline personality disorder.
C. Schizotypal personality disorder.
D. Schizoid personality disorder.
E. Avoidant personality disorder.

17.12 Which of the following personality disorders is associated with low resting pulse, low skin conductance, and increased amplitude on event-related potentials?

A. Antisocial personality disorder.
B. Borderline personality disorder.
C. Schizotypal personality disorder.
D. Schizoid personality disorder.
E. Avoidant personality disorder.

17.13 A 27-year-old software engineer seeks psychiatric treatment for anxiety. He has lived alone all his adult life. Outside of work, he has no social contacts apart from a weekly telephone call to his mother. He spends most of his free time playing video games, and he expresses little interest in developing more social relationships or having a romantic relationship. He does not endorse any symptoms of major depression or psychosis. He is very stiff and formal in interview and displays little emotion. Which of the following is the most likely diagnosis?

A. Avoidant personality disorder.
B. Schizotypal personality disorder.
C. Schizoid personality disorder.
D. Autism spectrum disorder.
E. Antisocial personality disorder.

17.14 You see a 33-year-old unemployed man in the outpatient clinic. He reports that he would like your assistance in getting disability for "anxiety." He says that for as long as he recalls, he has felt uncomfortable in social situations because he fears that other people will not understand him. He has never married and has no children. He has trouble maintaining employment because of anxiety. He sometimes thinks that magazine articles have special messages for him and may see shadows that look like people or animals. He has been trying to learn how to communicate telepathically by studying a "new age" book purchased on the Internet but has not been successful. He denies any history of auditory hallucinations and does not appear to have delusions. Which of the following is the most likely diagnosis?

A. Schizophrenia.
B. Schizotypal personality disorder.
C. Avoidant personality disorder.
D. Schizoid personality disorder.
E. Schizoaffective disorder.

17.15 Which of the following is *not* a trait of histrionic personality disorder?

A. Unease in situations in which one is not the center of attention.
B. Inappropriate sexually seductive or provocative behavior.
C. Rapidly shifting and shallow expression of emotions.
D. Transient, stress-related paranoid ideation or severe dissociative symptoms.
E. Self-dramatization, theatricality, and exaggerated expression of emotion.

17.16 A 26-year-old woman comes to your clinic to establish care for her mood swings that other psychiatrists have diagnosed as "bipolar disorder." She has persistent depression and severe mood swings, but she has never had a period of decreased sleep, pressured speech, or disinhibition that lasted for several days. She uses a razor blade to make small cuts on her forearms when anxious or upset but denies that she does this to kill herself. She has had several psychiatric hospitalizations for suicidal ideation, and she has overdosed multiple times. She endorses a deep fear that her loved ones will abandon her, and she has chronic feelings of emptiness. After your interview, she says that she thinks you are the best doctor she has ever had and that she has great confidence in your abilities. She speaks very poorly of her previous psychiatrist. Which of the following is the most likely diagnosis?

A. Bipolar II disorder.
B. Histrionic personality disorder.

C.  Borderline personality disorder.

D.  Dependent personality disorder.

E.  Schizotypal personality disorder.

17.17  Which of the following is *not* a recommended treatment for borderline personality disorder?

A.  Dialectical behavior therapy.

B.  Benzodiazepines for accompanying anxiety.

C.  Systems Training for Emotional Predictability and Problem Solving (STEPPS).

D.  Antipsychotic medications for perceptual distortions and anger dyscontrol.

E.  Selective serotonin reuptake inhibitors (SSRIs) for depression.

17.18  A 40-year-old business executive seeks treatment for depression. She reports being upset since a colleague was given a promotion that she feels was rightfully hers. Her long-term goal is to become the CEO of a major global corporation. During the session, she questions the therapist's credentials, and at one point she accuses the therapist of being envious of her superior social status. She does not return after the first session and later tells an acquaintance that it was because the therapist didn't give her the admiration that she deserves. Which of the following is the most likely diagnosis?

A.  Antisocial personality disorder.

B.  Borderline personality disorder.

C.  Narcissistic personality disorder.

D.  Dependent personality disorder.

E.  Histrionic personality disorder.

17.19  Avoidant personality disorder can be very difficult to distinguish from which of the following disorders?

A.  Social anxiety disorder.

B.  Generalized anxiety disorder.

C.  Panic disorder.

D.  Persistent depressive disorder.

E.  Autism spectrum disorder.

17.20 Ebenezer Scrooge comes to your practice seeking therapy for life dissatisfaction. He spends all his time working even though he is very wealthy. A cheerless man, he is reluctant to spend his money on basic amenities such as heating during the cold winter months. He has no social life and few recreational interests. He often rejects his nephew's dinner invitations. He expresses rigid, controversial opinions, such as that donating to charity is wasteful given that his hard-earned tax dollars finance workhouses and debtors' prisons. He micromanages his sole employee, but he reserves several tasks for himself for fear that his employee is not competent to handle these necessities to his satisfaction. Which of the following is the most likely diagnosis?

A. Schizoid personality disorder.
B. Narcissistic personality disorder.
C. Obsessive-compulsive personality disorder.
D. Avoidant personality disorder.
E. Antisocial personality disorder.

# — CHAPTER 18 —

# Psychiatric Emergencies

18.1 Aggressive behavior is associated with which of the following findings in the cerebrospinal fluid (CSF)?

A. Dopamine excess.
B. Norepinephrine excess.
C. Serotonin deficiency.
D. Acetylcholine deficiency.
E. Glutamine excess.

18.2 Which of the following is the single best predictor of future violent behavior?

A. Threats of violence.
B. Diagnosis of a severe mental illness (e.g., schizophrenia, bipolar disorder).
C. Previous psychiatric hospitalization.
D. Substance abuse history.
E. History of violence.

18.3 Which of the following personality disorders is most often associated with violent behavior?

A. Paranoid personality disorder.
B. Antisocial personality disorder.
C. Schizotypal personality disorder.
D. Narcissistic personality disorder.
E. Schizoid personality disorder.

18.4    Which of the following best describes the natural history of anti-social and borderline personality disorders?

A. Patients tend to act out more as they grow older.
B. Patients tend to act out less as they grow older.
C. Patients' tendency to act out does not change.
D. Patients only tend to act out less with age if they do not have a childhood history of conduct disorder.
E. Patients only tend to act out less with age if they do not have a childhood history of fire setting or cruelty to animals.

18.5    A psychiatrist is called to evaluate a patient in the emergency department whose chief complaint is homicidal ideation. The psychiatrist remains calm and speaks softly. She seats herself for the interview and allows distance between herself and the patient. She is careful to always make direct eye contact and to project empathy and concern. She asks nonjudgmental questions during the interview. Which of the following behaviors displayed by the psychiatrist is *not* recommended?

A. Speaking softly.
B. Sitting during the interview because psychiatrists should stand in order to be ready to escape.
C. Projecting empathy and concern because it can seem patronizing to a violent patient.
D. Use of direct eye contact.
E. Asking nonjudgmental questions.

18.6    You are seeing a patient with schizophrenia in the emergency department. The patient acknowledges his diagnosis and reports a worsening of symptoms. He reports that he has been hearing voices that have been telling him to kill a family member, something that he does not want to do. He has been hospitalized multiple times but does not have a history of violence. The patient is pleasant and cooperative. Which of the following is the most concerning risk factor for violence?

A. Lack of insight.
B. Stated desire to hurt or kill.
C. Presence of command hallucinations.
D. Diagnosis of panic disorder.
E. History of psychiatric hospitalization.

18.7 Which of the following combinations of medications is commonly given to calm acutely agitated patients?

A. Alprazolam and diphenhydramine.
B. Chlorpromazine and clonazepam.
C. Olanzapine and lorazepam.
D. Haloperidol and lorazepam.
E. Diphenhydramine and alprazolam.

18.8 Fill in the blank: Suicide is the _____ leading cause of death in persons between ages 15 and 24 years.

A. First.
B. Second.
C. Third.
D. Fifth.
E. Eleventh.

18.9 Which of the following is true regarding most people who commit suicide?

A. They usually do not tell anyone before committing suicide.
B. They may tell a friend or family member but usually do not seek medical help.
C. They usually communicate their suicidal intentions to and see physicians before they die.
D. They usually see a physician but do not usually tell their physician that they are having suicidal thoughts.
E. They usually do not have a primary care physician.

18.10 Which of the following individuals is probably at highest risk for completing suicide?

A. 25-year-old divorced African American man.
B. 55-year-old married white woman.
C. 60-year-old widowed white man.
D. 19-year-old single African American woman.
E. 40-year-old divorced white woman.

18.11 Which of the following is associated with a lower risk for suicide?

A. Major depression.
B. Male sex.

C. Hopelessness.
D. Substance use disorder.
E. African American race.

18.12  Suicide is associated with which of the following CSF findings?

A. Dopamine excess.
B. Norepinephrine excess.
C. Serotonin deficiency.
D. Acetylcholine deficiency.
E. Glutamine excess.

18.13  What is the most common method used to commit suicide in the United States?

A. Overdose.
B. Cutting.
C. Hanging.
D. Firearm.
E. Jumping.

18.14  Which of the following is one of the strongest correlates of suicidal behavior, independent of psychiatric diagnosis?

A. Presence of a mental illness.
B. History of violence.
C. Recent psychiatric hospitalization.
D. Hopelessness.
E. Psychosocial stressors.

18.15  For which group of patients is suicide frequently preceded by the loss of a relationship in the past year?

A. Alcoholic persons.
B. Patients with major depressive disorder.
C. Older patients with cognitive decline.
D. Adolescents with behavior problems.
E. People with a personality disorder.

18.16  What medications are associated with lowered rates of suicide?

A. Haloperidol.
B. Lithium.
C. Clozapine.
D. Options A and B.
E. Options B and C.

# ──CHAPTER 19──

# Legal Issues

19.1 Which of the following is a criminal and not a civil issue?

A. Determining whether to hospitalize a patient for acute homicidal ideation against his or her will.
B. Determining whether a patient with schizophrenia is capable of understanding court processes and assisting the court-appointed attorney.
C. Potential Health Insurance Portability and Accountability Act (HIPAA) violations.
D. Providing information about proposed treatments and alternatives and ensuring that the patient is capable of understanding these issues.
E. Determining whether a psychiatrist was negligent in his professional duties after abruptly terminating a doctor-patient relationship because the patient did not promptly pay a bill.

19.2 Which of the following is *not* a key criterion considered in civil commitment proceedings?

A. Mental illness.
B. Poor social support.
C. Dangerousness.
D. Inability to properly care for oneself.
E. "Grave disability."

19.3 What level of evidence is generally required in cases of civil commitment?

A. Beyond a reasonable doubt.
B. Clear and convincing evidence.

C. Preponderance of the evidence.

D. Substantial evidence.

E. Some credible evidence.

19.4 Most states have provisions for

A. Involuntary inpatient treatment only.

B. Involuntary outpatient treatment only.

C. Both involuntary inpatient and involuntary outpatient treatment.

D. Neither involuntary nor voluntary outpatient treatment.

E. Voluntary outpatient treatment only.

19.5 In which of the following situations is it the *least* clear cut whether patient confidentiality may be broken according to U.S. laws?

A. Reporting infectious disease such as tuberculosis or sexually transmitted infections.

B. Warning potential victims about threats made by patients.

C. Allowing access to medical charts for billing purposes.

D. Communicating with the family of a nonviolent psychiatric patient.

E. All the above are clear-cut cases in which confidentiality may be breached.

19.6 Which of the following are reasons that psychiatrists are sued for malpractice?

A. Failure to obtain informed consent.

B. Patient suicide.

C. Alleged injury from psychotropic medication.

D. Patient abandonment.

E. All the above.

19.7 What percentage of physicians will face at least one malpractice suit at some point during their careers?

A. 10%.

B. 35%.

C. 50%.

D. 65%.

E. 80%.

19.8 According to the American Psychiatric Association, at what point does it become acceptable for a psychiatrist to have an intimate relationship with a former patient?

A. 6 months after termination of the doctor-patient relationship.
B. 1 year after termination of the doctor-patient relationship.
C. 3 years after termination of the doctor-patient relationship.
D. 10 years after termination of the doctor-patient relationship.
E. Never.

19.9 In order to be competent to stand trial, a defendant must meet all the following criteria *except*

A. Being able to understand the nature of the charges against him or her.
B. Being able to understand the possible penalty.
C. Having been shown to have both bad behavior and blameworthy state of mind at the time of the offense.
D. Being able to understand the legal issues and procedures.
E. Being capable of working with an attorney in preparing the defense.

19.10 According to current U.S. laws, a crime occurs when

A. Illegal behavior occurs, regardless of the perpetrator's state of mind.
B. Illegal behavior occurs, and the perpetrator has a blameworthy state of mind.
C. A perpetrator has a blameworthy state of mind regardless of whether illegal behavior occurs.
D. Illegal behavior occurs, and the person does not have demonstrable mental illness.
E. A person with mental illness has a blameworthy state of mind.

19.11 Which of the following forms the basis of the insanity defense?

A. The *M'Naghten* standard.
B. The *Drummond* standard.
C. *Dusky v. United States*.
D. The *Tarasoff* rule.
E. The Peel Law.

19.12 A patient reveals to his psychiatrist that he plans to harm a neighbor. The psychiatrist is obligated to break confidentiality in order
to protect the potential victim. How shall the psychiatrist proceed?

A. Phone the neighbor to report the threat.
B. Phone the local police.
C. Ask the patient to phone the neighbor.
D. Report the threat to the local newspaper.
E. None of the above.

19.13 A woman with a psychosis is charged with murder. During her
pretrial screening, her speech is disorganized such that she cannot engage in coherent dialogue with her attorneys. Which of the
following best describes her legal situation regarding the charges
against her?

A. She is competent to stand trial but not guilty by reason of in-
sanity.
B. She is not competent to stand trial and not guilty by reason of
insanity.
C. She is not competent to stand trial, and whether she is not
guilty by reason of insanity has yet to be demonstrated.
D. She is guilty but mentally ill.
E. She has diminished capacity.

# CHAPTER 20

# Psychotherapy

20.1 In what form of therapy would the therapist offer praise, reassurance, and encouragement and give specific advice with the goal of helping the patient get through a difficult situation?

A. Cognitive-behavioral therapy.
B. Interpersonal psychotherapy.
C. Supportive psychotherapy.
D. Acceptance and commitment therapy.
E. Psychodynamic psychotherapy.

20.2 A therapist tells a patient who is afraid of elevators to ride an elevator continuously until his or her anxiety is gone. What is this technique called?

A. In vivo exposure
B. Imaginal exposure.
C. Behavioral activation.
D. Flooding.
E. Relaxation training.

20.3 Exposure, flooding, and relaxation training are techniques used in which form of psychotherapy?

A. Cognitive-behavioral therapy.
B. Behavior therapy.
C. Acceptance and commitment therapy.
D. Psychodynamic therapy.
E. Interpersonal psychotherapy.

20.4   What form of therapy has the goal of helping individuals adapt to the pain, grief, and inevitable disappointments that are part of life by developing greater psychological flexibility?

A. Supportive psychotherapy.
B. Cognitive-behavioral therapy.
C. Interpersonal psychotherapy.
D. Psychodynamic psychotherapy.
E. Acceptance and commitment therapy.

20.5   A therapist has a patient visualize being in an elevator to help him overcome his fear of elevators. This is an example of which of the following?

A. Relaxation training.
B. Imaginal exposure.
C. In vivo exposure.
D. Flooding.
E. Behavioral activation.

20.6   A therapist is working with a professional musician who has depression. The patient tells the therapist that she stopped playing the guitar 2 months earlier because it no longer brings her pleasure. She previously had been playing the guitar for several hours daily. The therapist proposes that she begin playing the guitar again every day, despite her lack of interest. This is an example of which of the following?

A. Relaxation training.
B. Imaginal exposure.
C. In vivo exposure.
D. Flooding.
E. Behavioral activation.

20.7   Which of the following is *not* part of Beck's cognitive triad of depression?

A. Negative view of oneself.
B. Negative view of relationships.
C. Negative view of the future.
D. Negative interpretation of experience.
E. More than one of the above.

20.8 Learning to correct automatic thoughts, schemas, and distortions is a key part of which kind of therapy?

A. Behavior therapy.
B. Cognitive-behavioral therapy.
C. Interpersonal therapy.
D. Psychodynamic psychotherapy.
E. Supportive psychotherapy.

20.9 An overzealous premedical student believes that she must get a perfect score on all of her assignments to have a chance of getting into medical school lest she be forced to spend the rest of her career working in the food service industry. This is an example of which of the following?

A. Overgeneralization.
B. Selective abstraction.
C. Dichotomous thinking.
D. Personalization.
E. Magnification and minimization.

20.10 A chess player wins three matches and loses one. He concludes that he got lucky in the three matches that he won and that he lost the other match because he is a terrible chess player. This is an example of which of the following?

A. Arbitrary inference.
B. Overgeneralization.
C. Dichotomous thinking.
D. Personalization.
E. Magnification and minimization.

20.11 A hard-working businesswoman arrives 30 minutes late to work because of an unexpected traffic jam caused by a car accident. She berates herself for her lack of responsibility and punctuality. This is an example of which of the following?

A. Arbitrary inference.
B. Overgeneralization.
C. Dichotomous thinking.
D. Personalization.
E. Magnification and minimization.

20.12 What is the most important component of relationship psycho-therapy?

A. The empathic and caring attitude of the therapist.
B. The neutrality of the therapist.
C. Reflection on early life experiences.
D. The correction of negative automatic thoughts and schemas.
E. Working on interpersonal disputes and deficits.

20.13 One of your patients is experiencing stress and anxiety that you attribute to coping with the new responsibilities that come with parenthood. Which type of psychotherapy would be especially suited to address this sort of problem?

A. Behavior therapy.
B. Cognitive-behavioral therapy.
C. Psychodynamic psychotherapy.
D. Interpersonal therapy.
E. Supportive therapy.

20.14 Which of the following is *not* one of the four domains of interpersonal therapy?

A. Grief.
B. Interpersonal disputes.
C. Acceptance and commitment.
D. Role transitions.
E. Interpersonal deficits.

20.15 A 26-year-old woman seeks treatment of her mood instability, difficult relationships, and self-harming behaviors. She is angry and irritable and says that previous therapists have not helped. She takes fluoxetine for her depression and anxiety, but it provides little symptomatic relief. She asks if there is something else you can do for her. Which of the following programs might be beneficial to her?

A. Dialectical behavior therapy (DBT).
B. Mentalization therapy.
C. Systems Training for Emotional Predictability and Problem Solving.
D. Schema-focused therapy.
E. All the above.

20.16 You are seeing a 23-year-old man with schizophrenia in your office. The patient does not have any active positive symptoms of psychosis but is awkward in interpersonal interactions and has difficulty with everyday tasks (e.g., maintaining appropriate hygiene). Which form of therapy would be beneficial in order to improve this patient's functional status?

A. Behavior therapy.
B. Cognitive-behavioral therapy.
C. Psychodynamic psychotherapy.
D. Interpersonal therapy.
E. Social skills training.

# — CHAPTER 21 —

# Somatic Treatments

21.1 What was the world's first antipsychotic?

A. Haloperidol.
B. Thioridazine.
C. Fluphenazine.
D. Chlorpromazine.
E. Trifluoperazine.

21.2 Compared with chlorpromazine, haloperidol

A. Has more anticholinergic side effects.
B. Is less sedating.
C. Causes fewer extrapyramidal side effects (EPS).
D. Is more likely to cause orthostatic hypotension.
E. Is associated with a much greater incidence of metabolic syndrome.

21.3 The potency of first-generation antipsychotic drugs correlates most closely with which of the following?

A. Affinity for 5-hydroxytryptamine (serotonin) type 2A (5-HT$_{2A}$) receptors.
B. Anticholinergic activity.
C. Antihistaminic activity.
D. Dopamine 2 (D$_2$) receptor affinity.
E. Noradrenergic receptor affinity.

21.4   As a general rule, most oral antipsychotics have a half-life of approximately

A. 1 hour.
B. 4 hours.
C. 12 hours.
D. 1 day.
E. 5 days.

21.5   Which of the cytochrome P450 (CYP) enzymes is involved in the metabolism of antipsychotic medications?

A. 2D6.
B. 1A2.
C. 3A4.
D. 2D6, 1A2, and 3A4.
E. Metabolism does not occur because they are renally excreted.

21.6   You are following a 21-year-old man with schizophrenia on an inpatient psychiatric unit. After 4 weeks, he remains floridly psychotic despite increasing doses of haloperidol, administered as oral tablets. His haloperidol blood level is 1 ng/mL. What does this suggest?

A. Psychotic symptoms are refractory to treatment with haloperidol.
B. The patient is a rapid metabolizer of haloperidol.
C. The patient is not swallowing the haloperidol tablets.
D. This blood level suggests laboratory error.
E. Haloperidol blood levels do not correlate with treatment response.

21.7   You are following a 21-year-old man with schizophrenia who has been hospitalized for 6 weeks. The patient continues to be floridly psychotic despite increasing doses of haloperidol, administered as oral tablets. His haloperidol blood level is 15 ng/mL. What does this suggest?

A. Psychotic symptoms are refractory to treatment with haloperidol.
B. The patient is a rapid metabolizer of haloperidol.
C. The patient is not swallowing the haloperidol tablets.

D. This blood level suggests laboratory error.

E. Haloperidol blood levels do not correlate with treatment response.

21.8 How long is an adequate trial of an antipsychotic drug?

A. 4–6 days.
B. 4–6 weeks.
C. 2–3 months.
D. 6–8 months.
E. The duration of an adequate trial depends on the specific agent.

21.9 What is the primary reason that clozapine is a second-line choice for treating psychosis?

A. Because many patients have refractory schizophrenia, clozapine is always in short supply.
B. Because clozapine can cause significant weight gain.
C. Because clozapine does not work as well as other antipsychotics for treating refractory symptoms.
D. Because clozapine can cause agranulocytosis, making it necessary for patients to have white blood cell counts checked regularly.
E. Because it takes 3–6 months to reach steady state.

21.10 You are seeing a 21-year-old man with schizophrenia in the outpatient clinic. His psychotic symptoms have been in remission on a moderate dose of haloperidol for the past 3 years. He has been admitted to the hospital three times for acute exacerbations of his psychosis but has never engaged in dangerous behaviors. He is in school and reports that he has a good mood. The patient is interested in discontinuing antipsychotic medications, even though he has tolerated the medication well. What is your recommendation?

A. "Now would be a good time for a trial without medications."
B. "We should make sure that you remain stable for another 2 years before attempting to discontinue medications."
C. "You should take the medication for the rest of your life."
D. "Let's try a new antipsychotic medication."
E. "Let's substitute a mild antidepressant for your other symptoms such as lack of motivation."

21.11 A patient with schizophrenia is admitted to an inpatient unit for acute psychosis, agitation, and violent ideation. He has had two recent (and similar) admissions, and he readily admits to not taking prescribed aripiprazole tablets because he believes that they are poisoned. His symptoms have responded well to antipsychotics when prescribed and monitored in the hospital. Which of the following is the best long-term strategy for managing the patient's symptoms?

A. Switch to a long-acting injectable antipsychotic.
B. Restart aripiprazole.
C. Switch to clozapine.
D. Switch to haloperidol.
E. Switch to risperidone.

21.12 You are seeing a 35-year-old woman with schizoaffective disorder in the outpatient clinic. The patient's psychotic symptoms have been well controlled on fluphenazine for the past several years. In interview, she displays abnormal involuntary movements of her mouth and tongue of which she is not aware. The movements are most consistent with which of the following?

A. Pseudoparkinsonism.
B. Akathisia.
C. Tardive dyskinesia.
D. Acute dystonic reaction.
E. Anticholinergic side effect.

21.13 A 19-year-old man recently started on haloperidol for schizophrenia comes to the clinic as a walk-in requesting to be seen urgently for "anxiety." The patient paces in the waiting room, is fidgety, and squirms in a chair during an interview. Which of the following best explains the patient's symptoms?

A. Akathisia.
B. Generalized anxiety disorder.
C. Mania.
D. Acute dystonic reaction.
E. Tardive dyskinesia.

21.14 A 42-year-old woman presents to the emergency department complaining of muscle stiffness. Her neck is twisted to the left, and she reports that she cannot move it. She was discharged from the inpatient psychiatric unit a day earlier after starting antipsychotic treatment for an acute psychosis. Which of the following is the best way to manage her symptoms?

A. Discontinue the antipsychotic.
B. Switch to a different antipsychotic.
C. Administer intramuscular benztropine or diphenhydramine.
D. Administer oral propranolol.
E. Administer oral clonidine.

21.15 Which of the following is *not* an anticholinergic adverse effect of antipsychotics?

A. Diarrhea.
B. Urinary retention.
C. Blurry vision.
D. Dry mouth.
E. Exacerbation of narrow-angle glaucoma.

21.16 Regular monitoring of body mass index (BMI), blood pressure, fasting glucose, and lipid panels is recommended for patients who are taking which of the following?

A. Haloperidol.
B. Risperidone.
C. Venlafaxine.
D. Sertraline.
E. Nortriptyline.

21.17 A 45-year-old woman who takes haloperidol for her schizophrenia is admitted to a medical unit for rigidity, high fever, and mental status changes. Laboratory tests show elevated creatinine phosphokinase and liver enzymes. What is the most important aspect of acute care for this patient?

A. Start dantrolene.
B. Start bromocriptine.

C. Start electroconvulsive therapy (ECT).

D. Stop haloperidol and provide supportive care.

E. Transfer to psychiatric inpatient unit.

21.18 You are treating a 35-year-old man for a major depressive disorder and narcissistic personality disorder. He demands that he receive the most effective antidepressant available. What do you do?

A. Prescribe levomilnacipran because it is one of the newer antidepressants.

B. Prescribe escitalopram because it is a standard selective serotonin reuptake inhibitor (SSRI).

C. Prescribe venlafaxine because of its dual action in targeting norepinephrine and serotonin neurotransmission.

D. Advise him that antidepressants are—for the most part—equally effective.

E. Recommend psychotherapy to address his underlying narcissism.

21.19 Which type of depression is expected to respond best to an antidepressant?

A. Persistent depressive disorder (dysthymia).

B. Atypical depression.

C. Major depressive disorder with comorbid hypochondriasis.

D. Major depressive disorder with comorbid somatic symptom disorder.

E. Major depressive disorder with melancholic features.

21.20 Which SSRI has the longest half-life?

A. Fluoxetine.

B. Sertraline.

C. Citalopram.

D. Escitalopram.

E. Paroxetine.

21.21 Which of the following is *not* a typical SSRI adverse effect?

A. Loose bowel movements.

B. Anxiety.

C. Sexual dysfunction.

D. Nausea.

E. Orthostatic hypotension.

21.22 You prescribe citalopram to a 28-year-old man for obsessive-compulsive disorder. At follow-up, he reports that his symptoms have greatly improved, but he has developed delayed ejaculation that interferes with a new relationship. Which pharmacological strategy has *not* been recommended to address this problem?

A. Switch to bupropion.

B. Add bupropion to the citalopram.

C. Switch to duloxetine.

D. Take lorazepam prior to sexual activity.

E. Take sildenafil prior to sexual activity.

21.23 A 55-year-old woman is brought to the emergency department with an altered mental status, flushing, diaphoresis, and myoclonic jerks. She was recently started on a third antidepressant for treatment-refractory depression. Which of the following is the most likely diagnosis?

A. Catatonia.

B. Serotonin syndrome.

C. NMS.

D. SSRI discontinuation syndrome.

E. Acute dystonic reaction.

21.24 Which antidepressant is contraindicated for a 45-year-old man with epilepsy?

A. Venlafaxine.

B. Mirtazapine.

C. Trazodone.

D. Bupropion.

E. Desvenlafaxine.

21.25 Which of the following patients is a good candidate for a trial of duloxetine?

A. A 37-year-old woman with a history of multiple recent overdose attempts.

B. A 60-year-old man with chronic depression and alcoholism.

C. A 20-year-old man with depression, posttraumatic stress disorder, and insomnia.

D. A 54-year-old woman with depression partially controlled by an MAOI.

E. A 48-year-old man with major depressive disorder and neuropathic pain from diabetes mellitus.

21.26 Which of the following antidepressants is the best choice for a 30-year-old man with a first episode of major depressive disorder with melancholic features including insomnia and weight loss?

A. Citalopram.
B. Bupropion.
C. Duloxetine.
D. Mirtazapine.
E. Venlafaxine.

21.27 Which of the following antidepressants is widely used off-label to treat insomnia?

A. Venlafaxine.
B. Duloxetine.
C. Trazodone.
D. Phenelzine.
E. Sertraline.

21.28 A 35-year-old man who has treatment-refractory depression presents to the emergency department because of a prolonged painful erection. The patient has been taking multiple psychotropic medications to treat his disorder, including sertraline, bupropion, buspirone, trazodone, and lithium. Which medication is most likely to have caused his condition?

A. Sertraline.
B. Bupropion.
C. Buspirone.
D. Trazodone.
E. Lithium.

21.29 What is the mechanism of action of the antidepressant vilazodone?

A. It selectively inhibits reuptake of serotonin.
B. It inhibits reuptake of both serotonin and norepinephrine.

C. It is a dopamine $D_2$ receptor antagonist.

D. It is a serotonin reuptake inhibitor and 5-$HT_{1A}$ receptor partial agonist.

E. It blocks 5-$HT_2$ receptors and weakly inhibits serotonin reuptake.

21.30 Which of the following tricyclic antidepressants has an established therapeutic blood level range?

A. Amitriptyline.

B. Nortriptyline.

C. Doxepin.

D. Clomipramine.

E. Protriptyline.

21.31 Why are MAOIs not more widely used to treat depression?

A. Because of the required long washout period when transitioning a patient to or from an MAOI to avoid serotonin syndrome.

B. Because a hypertensive crisis could result if an MAOI is combined with foods that contain tyramine.

C. Because they are potent α-adrenergic blockers and can cause orthostatic hypotension.

D. Because patients prescribed MAOIs should carry a list of prohibited foods, wear a medical bracelet indicating that they take an MAOI, and carry a 10-mg tablet of nifedipine with them at all times.

E. All the above.

21.32 What is a reasonable length for an adequate trial of an antidepressant?

A. 3–5 days.

B. 3–5 weeks.

C. 1–2 months.

D. 3–4 months.

E. It depends on the agent.

21.33 A 25-year-old man with a well-established diagnosis of bipolar I disorder presents to the emergency department, having been brought in by the police for disruptive behavior. He has not been sleeping for the past 3 days, and he believes that he is Jesus Christ. He is very agitated, and you believe that he is potentially dangerous. Which of the following medications would be most effective in calming him while in the emergency department?

A. Lithium.
B. Valproate.
C. Lamotrigine.
D. Haloperidol.
E. Carbamazepine.

21.34 Which of the following medications has been shown to reduce suicidal behavior?

A. Valproate.
B. Lithium.
C. Carbamazepine.
D. Lamotrigine.
E. Alprazolam.

21.35 Which of the following is *not* an appropriate use of lithium?

A. Prophylaxis of manic episodes in bipolar I patients.
B. Reducing the severity of manic episodes.
C. Adjunctive treatment to prevent recurrences of depression in patients with unipolar major depressive disorder.
D. Achieving rapid sedation of an acutely agitated manic patient.
E. Prophylaxis of depressive episodes in patients with a bipolar disorder.

21.36 When is the best time to check a lithium blood level?

A. 8 hours after the last dose for a manic patient and 18 hours after the last dose for a euthymic patient.
B. 12 hours after the last dose.
C. 8 hours after the last dose.
D. 18 hours after the last dose.
E. Accurate lithium levels can be obtained at any time because the elimination half-life of lithium is 36 hours.

21.37 Which mood-stabilizing agent does *not* undergo mostly hepatic metabolism?

A. Valproate.
B. Lamotrigine.
C. Lithium.
D. Carbamazepine.
E. None of the above.

21.38 Which mood-stabilizing agent can in rare cases cause Stevens-Johnson syndrome?

A. Valproate.
B. Lamotrigine.
C. Lithium.
D. Carbamazepine.
E. Aripiprazole.

21.39 For which of the following cases is lamotrigine monotherapy most appropriate?

A. A patient with bipolar I disorder and a history of multiple hospitalizations for mania and a history of nonresponse to lithium.
B. A patient with bipolar I disorder with a history of multiple hospitalizations for mania and a history of response to lithium.
C. A patient with bipolar I disorder who presents with irritable mania.
D. A patient with bipolar I disorder with mixed mania and depression.
E. A patient with bipolar I disorder with several severe depressive episodes and infrequent manic episodes.

21.40 Which patient with bipolar I disorder is a good candidate for carbamazepine therapy?

A. A patient with irritable mania who has not responded to lithium.
B. A patient in a mixed episode.
C. A patient with more than four mood episodes per year who has not responded to lithium.

D. A patient with mostly depressed episodes and mild infrequent hypomanic episodes.

E. None of the above.

21.41 Which neurotransmitter is intimately involved in the mechanism of action for benzodiazepines?

A. Glutamate.

B. Norepinephrine.

C. Gabapentin.

D. γ-Aminobutyric acid (GABA).

E. Serotonin.

21.42 Benzodiazepines are remarkably versatile drugs. These medications are used to treat all of the following *except*

A. Seizure disorders.

B. Anxiety.

C. Alcohol withdrawal.

D. Sleep disorders.

E. Major depressive disorder.

21.43 Which of the following medications has an FDA indication for the treatment of generalized anxiety disorder?

A. Buspirone.

B. Bupropion.

C. Alprazolam.

D. Aripiprazole.

E. None of the above.

21.44 Extrapyramidal syndromes have been treated with all of the following medications *except*

A. Propranolol.

B. Diphenhydramine.

C. Amantadine.

D. Benztropine.

E. Trazodone.

21.45 Which of the following conditions represents an absolute contra-indication to administering ECT?

A. Recent myocardial infarction.
B. Unstable coronary artery disease.
C. Space-occupying brain lesions.
D. Venous thrombosis.
E. Chronically low platelet count.

21.46 A 36-year-old woman is receiving ECT for treatment of her major depressive disorder. What should she be told about possible adverse effects of the treatment?

A. She might have permanent memory loss that will be most dense around the time of treatment.
B. She will have no memory loss because the psychiatrist will use unilateral lead placement.
C. She will have permanent memory loss that will mainly involve new memories following the conclusion of the treatment.
D. She will have no memory loss because the psychiatrist will use the minimal amount of electricity needed to be therapeutic.
E. None of the above.

STUDY GUIDE

PART II

# ANSWER GUIDE

# — CHAPTER 1 —

# Diagnosis and Classification

1.1    Which of the following terms is used to describe collections of symptoms that tend to co-occur and appear to have a characteristic course and outcome?

A. Disease.
B. Symptomatology.
C. Syndrome.
D. Pathophysiology.
E. Illness.

**The correct response is option C: Syndrome.**

Most of the disorders or diseases diagnosed in psychiatry are *syndromes*: collections of symptoms that tend to co-occur and appear to have a characteristic course and outcome. **(p. 3)**

1.2    Which of the following is *not* a clinical reason to diagnose patients?

A. To reduce the complexity of clinical phenomena.
B. To provide the patient a label with which to identify.
C. To facilitate communication among clinicians.
D. To predict the course of illness.
E. To determine treatment options.

**The correct response is option B: To provide the patient a label with which to identify.**

There are many reasons to diagnose patients. Diagnoses in psychiatry serve a variety of important purposes and are not just a

125

"label" (option B). Making a careful diagnosis is as fundamental in psychiatry as it is in the rest of medicine. Diagnoses introduce order and structure to our thinking and reduce the complexity of clinical phenomena (option A). Diagnoses facilitate communication among clinicians (option C). The use of diagnostic categories gives clinicians a kind of "shorthand" through which they can summarize large quantities of information relatively easily. Diagnoses help to predict outcome, are often used to choose an appropriate treatment (option E), and are used to assist in the search for pathophysiology and etiology (option D). **(pp. 4–6)**

1.3    Which DSM edition first provided specific diagnostic criteria for mental disorders?

A. DSM-I.
B. DSM-II.
C. DSM-III.
D. DSM-IV.
E. DSM-5.

**The correct response is option C: DSM-III.**

DSM-III—published in 1980—was transformative in part because of the introduction of diagnostic criteria sets. This addition helped change the way psychiatrists and other mental health professionals go about the diagnostic process. Definitions in DSM-I (1952) and DSM-II (1968) were brief, narrative descriptions that did not adequately fulfill many of the purposes for making a diagnosis. The authors of DSM-III agreed to formulate diagnostic criteria that would be as objective as possible to define each of the disorders and to base their decisions about defining criteria and overall organizational structure on existing research data whenever possible. **(p. 7)**

1.4    Which of the following is *not* an advantage of the DSM system?

A. It has substantially improved reliability of diagnoses.
B. It has substantially improved validity of diagnoses.
C. It has clarified the diagnostic process and history taking.
D. It has clarified and facilitated the process of differential diagnosis.
E. All the above are advantages of the DSM system.

**The correct response is option B: It has substantially improved validity of diagnoses.**

DSM has improved the *reliability* (option A) of diagnoses (i.e., that clinicians will give the same patient the same diagnosis for the same symptoms). DSM has also clarified the diagnostic process, history taking, and differential diagnosis through its emphasis on diagnostic criteria (options C, D). In contrast, *validity* (option B) refers to the ability of a diagnosis to predict prognosis, effective treatment, and, ultimately, etiology. Some have asserted that the DSM system has sacrificed validity on the altar of reliability. **(pp. 8–10)**

1.5    You are asked to evaluate a 55-year-old man on a general medical floor. You determine that he is delirious because of a hepatic encephalopathy. You learn that he drinks large quantities of distilled spirits daily and smokes one pack of cigarettes per day. Considering the *International Classification of Diseases* (ICD) and DSM rules, how would you record his diagnoses (i.e., in order of importance)?

    A. Delirium (principal diagnosis), alcohol use disorder, tobacco use disorder.
    B. Delirium due to hepatic encephalopathy (principal diagnosis), alcohol use disorder, tobacco use disorder.
    C. Alcohol use disorder (provisional diagnosis), delirium due to hepatic encephalopathy, tobacco use disorder.
    D. Hepatic encephalopathy, delirium due to hepatic encephalopathy (principal diagnosis), alcohol use disorder, tobacco use disorder.
    E. Delirium due to hepatic encephalopathy, hepatic encephalopathy, alcohol use disorder, tobacco use disorder.

**The correct response is option D: Hepatic encephalopathy, delirium due to hepatic encephalopathy (principal diagnosis), alcohol use disorder, tobacco use disorder.**

In DSM-5, diagnoses are ranked in order of their focus of attention or treatment, listing the condition chiefly responsible for a patient's hospital stay (or outpatient clinic visit) as the *principal diagnosis* (or *reason for visit*), which may be written parenthetically after the diagnosis (e.g., "[principal diagnosis]"). The only exception is that—according to the arcane coding rules in the

ICD system—if the mental disorder results from a medical condition, that medical condition is listed first. For example, if an outpatient with HIV disease seeks care for symptoms related to a mild neurocognitive disorder caused by the HIV, "HIV infection" is listed first, followed by "mild neurocognitive disorder due to HIV infection (reason for visit)." **(p. 12)**

1.6     You are evaluating a patient in the emergency department who you believe is likely experiencing a psychotic manic episode (bipolar I disorder with psychotic features). The patient is a poor historian, and you are not currently able to obtain collateral information to confirm the diagnosis. According to DSM, how should you document the diagnosis to reflect your uncertainty?

A. Rule out bipolar I disorder.
B. Evaluate for bipolar I disorder.
C. Bipolar I disorder versus psychosis not otherwise specified.
D. Bipolar I disorder (provisional).
E. Bipolar I disorder.

**The correct response is option D: Bipolar I disorder (provisional).**

If the clinician does not have sufficient information to allow a firm diagnosis, uncertainty may be indicated by recording "(provisional)" following the diagnosis (option D). **(p. 12)**

1.7     You are seeing a 25-year-old woman in the outpatient clinic for a routine follow-up visit. Major problems reported at the visit include stormy interpersonal relationships and frequent anger outbursts. You conclude that these symptoms result from her borderline personality disorder. The patient's symptoms also meet criteria for generalized anxiety disorder, and she smokes 10 cigarettes daily. How would you record the diagnoses according to DSM-5?

A. Axis I: generalized anxiety disorder, tobacco use disorder; Axis II: borderline personality disorder (principal diagnosis).
B. Borderline personality disorder (principal diagnosis), generalized anxiety disorder, tobacco use disorder.
C. Generalized anxiety disorder, borderline personality disorder, tobacco use disorder.
D. Tobacco use disorder, borderline personality disorder, generalized anxiety disorder.

E. Borderline personality disorder (provisional), generalized anxiety disorder, tobacco use disorder.

**The correct response is option B: Borderline personality disorder (principal diagnosis), generalized anxiety disorder, tobacco use disorder.**

The principal diagnosis should be listed first, followed by the other diagnoses. The phrase "(principal diagnosis)" or "(reason for visit)" can be used to indicate the primary diagnosis for which the patient is seeking care. The phrase "(provisional)" is used to show that a clinician is not certain about a diagnosis, but in this vignette the clinician is confident of the diagnosis of borderline personality disorder (option E). DSM-5 no longer uses the multiaxial system for diagnoses (option A). **(p. 12)**

1.8 A 34-year-old woman comes to your office for new-onset depression. The history reveals that along with depression, she has developed cold intolerance, fatigue, and weight gain. Routine laboratory testing reveals hypothyroidism, which you believe is the cause of her depression. What is the correct way to record the diagnoses?

A. Major depressive disorder (principal diagnosis), hypothyroidism.
B. Depression due to hypothyroidism (principal diagnosis), hypothyroidism.
C. Hypothyroidism, depression due to hypothyroidism (provisional).
D. Hypothyroidism, depression due to hypothyroidism (principal diagnosis).
E. Hypothyroidism, major depressive disorder (principal diagnosis).

**The correct response is option D: Hypothyroidism, depression due to hypothyroidism (principal diagnosis).**

According to ICD rules, if a mental disorder is caused by a physical condition, the physical condition should be listed first. In order to clarify that the patient is primarily seeking care for depression, the phrase "(principal diagnosis)" should be written after "depression due to hypothyroidism." Option B is incorrect because hypothyroidism should be the first diagnosis listed. Options A and E are incorrect because the question indicates that the depression is caused by hypothyroidism, rather than being an independent major depressive disorder diagnosis. Option C incorrectly uses the phrase "(provisional)." "(Provisional)" is used to indicate that the clinician does not have sufficient information to make a firm diagnosis, and the question stem does not indicate that there were any barriers to obtaining complete information. **(p. 12)**

1.9 Which of the following is not included in DSM-5?

A. Comorbidity.
B. Diagnostic features.
C. Treatment guidelines.
D. Suicide risk.
E. Risk and prognostic factors.

**The correct response is option C: Treatment guidelines.**

DSM-5 does not contain treatment guidelines (option C). DSM-5 contains information about diagnostic features, risk and prognostic factors, comorbidity, suicide risk, and all the other categories listed in Table 1–2, "Useful information in DSM-5 regarding each diagnosis." **(pp. 13–14)**

# — CHAPTER 2 —

# Interviewing and Assessment

2.1 A psychiatrist asks a patient to recall a list of three objects ("orange, airplane, tobacco") after 5 minutes. What type of memory does this test?

A. Ultrashort-term memory.
B. Very-short-term memory.
C. Short-term memory.
D. Medium-term memory.
E. Long-term memory.

**The correct response is option C: Short-term memory.**

Short-term memory is assessed by asking patients to recall a list of three objects after a delay of 3–5 minutes (option C). Very-short-term memory, or registration, is the patient's ability to immediately recall items after he or she is told them (option B). Long-term memory is assessed by asking the patient to recall events that occurred in the more remote past (option E). Ultrashort- and medium-term memory are not memory types (options A, D). **(p. 22)**

2.2 A psychiatrist asks a patient to tell her what the phrase "don't cry over spilled milk" means. The patient replies, "Milk isn't worth crying over because it's easy to come by." What does the patient's answer suggest?

A. Illogicality.
B. Poor abstraction.
C. Derailment.

D. Circumstantiality.

E. Poverty of content of speech.

**The correct response is option B: Poor abstraction.**

Proverb interpretation tests a patient's ability to think in the abstract. The patient in this example interprets the proverb literally, thus showing poor abstraction (option B). Derailment (option C) is when the patient has a pattern of spontaneous speech in which the ideas slip off the track onto another that is clearly but obliquely related or onto one completely unrelated. Illogicality (option A) refers to drawing conclusions that do not follow logically. Circumstantiality (option D) is a pattern of speech that is very indirect and delayed in reaching its goals. Poverty of content of speech (option E) is when the patient has adequate amount of speech but conveys little information. **(pp. 23, 37–39, 41)**

2.3 A man believes he is preventing cancer and maximizing his health by taking an expensive but otherwise innocuous herbal supplement. If asked, he will discuss the supplement with great interest but dismisses evidence that does not confirm his beliefs. Otherwise, this interest in the supplement has no significant influence on his day-to-day life. Which of the following terms best describes the man's beliefs?

A. Overvalued ideation.

B. Delusion.

C. Poor abstraction.

D. Impaired fund of knowledge.

E. Illogicality.

**The correct response is option A: Overvalued ideation.**

An overvalued idea is a false belief that is held with less than a delusional intensity (option A). Delusions (option B) are more intense and fixed than overvalued ideas, and they cannot be explained by a patient's cultural background. Ability for abstraction (option C) is part of the mental status examination, and it is sometimes assessed with proverb interpretation. Nothing in the vignette suggests that the man has an impaired fund of knowledge (option D). Illogicality (option E) refers to drawing conclusions that do not follow logically. **(pp. 23, 29, 38)**

2.4 A patient admits to her psychiatrist that she sometimes worries that events she reads about in magazines indirectly comment on her personal life. For example, one of her favorite magazines had a recipe for banana cream pie, which made her think that somehow the editor knew that this was her favorite pie. The psychiatrist asks her if she really believes this, and the patient reports that sometimes it does seem "silly." What term best describes the woman's suspicion?

A. Illogicality.
B. Persecutory delusions.
C. Delusions of reference.
D. Ideas of reference.
E. Thought broadcasting.

**The correct response is option D: Ideas of reference.**

*Ideas of reference* or *delusions of reference* are terms that describe when a patient believes that insignificant remarks, statements, or events have some special meaning for him or her. This patient is experiencing ideas of reference (option D) rather than delusions of reference (option C) because she can recognize that her ideas may not be true. People with persecutory delusions (option B) believe that they are being conspired against or persecuted in some way. Illogicality (option A) refers to drawing conclusions that do not follow logically. Thought broadcasting (option E) is when a patient believes that his or her thoughts are broadcast so that he or she or others can hear them. **(pp. 29–32, 38)**

2.5 A 35-year-old woman reports to her psychiatrist that, as part of a government conspiracy, a mind control device was implanted in her brain. She believes that the FBI (or possibly the CIA) is using this device to spy on her. Furthermore, she says that the device can control her body movements, making her feel like a puppet on a string. She describes how the device can remove thoughts from her brain like a vacuum cleaner while implanting thoughts that are not hers. Which of the following symptoms is *not* consistent with this patient's delusional system?

A. Delusions of passivity.
B. Thought withdrawal.
C. Thought insertion.

D. Somatic delusions.

E. Persecutory delusions.

**The correct response is option D: Somatic delusions.**

Somatic delusions (option D) occur when a patient believes that somehow his or her body is diseased, abnormal, or changed. This patient has a persecutory delusion (option E) that an implanted device is spying on her. The belief that the device controls her body is best described as a delusion of passivity (option A). The device can insert and delete her thoughts; this is called thought insertion (option C) and thought withdrawal (option B), respectively. **(pp. 29–33)**

2.6   A psychiatrist asks a patient where she lives. She replies, "I live in Springfield. It will be spring in another couple of months, but at least this winter has been mild. The winter tends to be pretty bad in Atlanta, which is where I lived until I moved to Springfield, but birds fly south in the winter. I'd really like to go to the beach just now." What is this an example of?

A. Tangentiality.

B. Circumstantiality.

C. Incoherence.

D. Illogicality.

E. Derailment.

**The correct response is option E: Derailment.**

Derailment (option E) is a pattern of spontaneous speech in which the ideas slip off the track onto another that is clearly but obliquely related or onto one completely unrelated. This is not tangentiality (option A) because when a patient exhibits tangentiality, the initial answer to the question is tangential or irrelevant. Circumstantiality (option B) is speech that is indirect and delayed in reaching its goal ideas. Incoherence (option C) refers to disorganization that occurs at the level of sentences rather than at the level of the overall stream of speech. Illogicality (option D) refers to drawing conclusions that do not follow logically. **(pp. 36–39)**

2.7   A psychiatrist asks a patient if he enjoyed his own birthday party the prior week. The patient responds by laboriously describing preparations for the party and then going into minute detail about the party, including minutiae such as the order of arrival of the guests and vivid descriptions of the appetizers. Ten minutes into this story, the psychiatrist realizes that the patient has not yet answered his question. What is this an example of?

A. Circumstantiality.
B. Pressured speech.
C. Derailment.
D. Tangentiality.
E. Distractible speech.

**The correct response is option A: Circumstantiality.**

Circumstantiality (option A) is speech that is indirect and delayed in reaching its goal ideas, which is the cardinal feature of the patient's story. This is not derailment because the content is on topic and logically connected (option C). This is not tangentiality because the patient is answering the question on topic (option D). Pressured speech is rapid and difficult to interrupt, with an increase in the overall amount of spontaneous speech. This story can be described as long-winded, but no further details are given to allow us to determine whether the speech is pressured (option B). Distractible speech (option E) occurs when the patient stops talking in the middle of a sentence or an idea and changes the subject in response to a nearby stimulus. **(pp. 37–40)**

2.8    A psychiatrist asks a patient where she lives. She replies, "I live in Springfield. The weather in spring makes me want to spring forth with joy. I like to drink fresh spring water. You need springs to build several different kinds of machines. Spring. Bring. Cling. Ring." What is the best way to describe this type of formal thought disorder?

A. Incoherence.
B. Clanging.
C. Distractible speech.
D. Pressured speech.
E. Alogia.

**The correct response is option B: Clanging.**

With clanging (option B), sounds rather than meaningful relationships among words appear to govern word choice, so that the intelligibility of the speech is impaired and redundant words are introduced in addition to rhyming relationships. This pattern of speech also may include punning associations, so that a word similar in sound brings in a new thought. With incoherence (option A), the relationship between sounds and word choice is not necessarily present. Distractible speech (option C) occurs when the patient stops talking in the middle of a sentence or an idea and changes the subject in response to a nearby stimulus. Pressured speech (option D) is rapid and difficult to interrupt. Alogia (option E) is a general term that describes impoverished thinking and cognition that is common in psychotic patients. **(pp. 38–41)**

2.9    A psychiatrist is interviewing a manic patient. The patient speaks very rapidly, and it is very difficult for the psychiatrist to get a word in. The patient is unable to adequately answer many routine questions because he is distracted by objects in the room such as chairs, the psychiatrist's identification badge, and the clock on the wall. Which of the following options best describes the patient's speech?

A. Pressured speech.
B. Distractible speech.
C. Both pressured speech and distractible speech.
D. Catatonic excitement.
E. Circumstantiality.

**The correct response is option C: Both pressured speech and distractible speech.**

The patient's speech is both pressured and distractible because it is rapid and difficult to interrupt, and he is unable to answer questions adequately because he is distracted by environmental stimuli (option C). With pressured speech, the patient has an increase in the amount of spontaneous speech compared with what is considered ordinary or socially customary. The patient talks rapidly and is difficult to interrupt (option A). Pressured speech is often seen in mania but can be found in other syndromes as well. Some sentences may be left uncompleted because of eagerness to get on to a new idea. Speech tends to be loud and emphatic. With distractible speech, however, the patient may stop talking in the middle of a sentence or an idea and changes the subject in response to a nearby stimulus, such as an object on a desk and the interviewer's clothing or appearance (option B). An example follows:

Subject: Then I left San Francisco and moved to…where did you get that tie? It looks like it's left over from the '50s. I like the warm weather in San Diego. Is that a conch shell on your desk? Have you ever gone scuba diving?

Catatonic excitement (option D) is when a patient has purposeless and stereotyped excited motor activity not influenced by external stimuli. Circumstantiality (option E) is speech that is indirect and delayed in reaching its goal ideas. **(pp. 39–40)**

2.10 In response to a routine question, a patient begins to answer appropriately but stops talking midsentence and stares off into space for 15 seconds. She then asks the interviewer to repeat the question. What does this exemplify?

A. Poverty of speech.
B. Poverty of content of speech.
C. Circumstantiality.
D. Perseveration.
E. Thought blocking.

**The correct response is option E: Thought blocking.**

Thought blocking (option E) describes when a patient's train of speech is interrupted before completion. Poverty of speech (option A) is a restricted amount of spontaneous speech, so that replies to questions tend to be brief, concrete, and unelaborated. Poverty of content of speech (option B) is when speech is adequate in amount but conveys little information. Perseveration (option D) is persistent repetition of words, ideas, or phrases by the patient. Circumstantiality (option C) is speech that is indirect and delayed in reaching its goal ideas. **(pp. 39, 41–42)**

2.11 A psychiatrist asks a patient where she lives. She replies, "I lived in Springfield many years ago." What is the best way to describe this formal thought disorder?

A. Tangentiality.
B. Circumstantiality.

C. Incoherence.
D. Illogicality.
E. Derailment.

**The correct response is option A: Tangentiality.**

Tangentiality is when a patient answers a direct question with an oblique, tangential, or irrelevant reply (option A). This contrasts with derailment (option E) when a patient will answer the question but quickly slip off the tracks to discuss matters that are obliquely related or completely unrelated to the original question. The two terms are not mutually exclusive. Circumstantiality (option B) refers to overly detailed speech that is delayed in reaching its goal. Incoherent speech (option C) is speech that has disorganized sentence structure such that it is incomprehensible. Illogical speech (option D) contains logical fallacies such as non sequiturs. **(pp. 37–39)**

2.12 A psychiatrist asks a patient where she lives. She replies, "I live in Springfield. In Springfield. That's where I live in Springfield."

A. Tangentiality.
B. Perseveration.
C. Incoherence.
D. Illogicality.
E. Derailment.

**The correct response is option B: Perseveration.**

In perseveration (option B), the patient consistently repeats words, phrases, or ideas. Tangentiality (option A) is when a patient answers a direct question with an oblique, tangential, or irrelevant reply. Incoherent speech (option C) is speech that has disorganized sentence structure such that it is incomprehensible. Illogical speech (option D) contains logical fallacies such as non sequiturs. Derailment (option E) is when a patient answers a question and then slips off the tracks to begin speaking about obliquely related or unrelated matters. **(pp. 37, 38, 42)**

2.13 A psychiatrist notes that a depressed patient is very slow to answer questions and that his speech and body movements are slow. Despite the slowness, the patient is fully aware of the situation and can answer questions appropriately. What is the correct term for this symptom?

A. Stupor.
B. Psychomotor retardation.
C. Psychomotor agitation.
D. Thought blocking.
E. Poverty of speech.

**The correct response is option B: Psychomotor retardation.**

Psychomotor retardation (option B) occurs when a depressed patient feels slowed down and experiences great difficulty moving. Psychomotor slowing is often found in major depression, but it is only one of many depressive symptoms. Stupor (option A) is a marked decrease in reactivity to the environment and a reduction of spontaneous movements and activity and is typically part of a catatonic syndrome. Psychomotor agitation (option C) is when the patient is unable to sit still and has a need to keep moving, which is the opposite of what is described in the vignette. Thought blocking (option D) is when patients lose track of their thoughts before their completion. Poverty of speech (option E) refers to a restricted amount of spontaneous speech. Replies tend to be monosyllabic, with some questions left unanswered altogether. **(pp. 40–42, 49–50)**

2.14 A patient reports to his psychiatrist that he has a fear of losing control and stabbing his 10-year-old son. He finds the thoughts very distressing. To ally his fears, he had his wife lock up all knives. What type of symptom has the man described to his doctor?

A. Specific phobia.
B. Delusion of guilt.
C. Compulsion.
D. Obsession.
E. Aggressive behavior.

**The correct response is option D: Obsession.**

Obsession (option D) is a persistent thought, impulse, or image that is unwanted and experienced as unpleasant, which is what the patient describes in the vignette. Even though he had his wife lock up the knives, his fear is not with the object itself, as in a specific phobia (option A), but with the thought that he might lose control. He might feel guilty about the thought, but it is not a delusion because he has not expressed a belief that he has done something unforgivable, such as stabbing his child (option B). Option C is not correct, because a compulsion is the behavioral response to an obsession—for example, checking something repeatedly. Option E is incorrect because the man has not shown any aggression toward the child. **(pp. 30, 36, 52–53)**

# — CHAPTER 3 —

# Neurobiology and Genetics of Mental Illness

3.1 Which of the following is *not* a primary function of the prefrontal system?

A. Mediation of attention and perception.
B. Mediation of affect and emotion.
C. Fear processing.
D. Temporal sequencing of behavior.
E. Moral judgment.

**The correct response is option C: Fear processing.**

Fear processing is associated with the limbic system, especially the amygdala (option C). Options A, B, D, and E are primary functions of the prefrontal system. This huge association region in the brain integrates input from much of the neocortex, limbic regions, hypothalamic and brain stem regions, and (via the thalamus) most of the rest of the brain. Its high degree of development in human beings suggests that it may mediate a variety of specifically human functions often referred to as *executive functions*. Lesion and trauma studies, supplemented by experimental studies in nonhuman primates, support the role of the prefrontal system in mediation of affect and emotion, mediation of attention and perception, the temporal sequencing of behavior, and moral judgment. **(pp. 57–59)**

3.2 Which of the following areas of the brain have a high concentration of dopamine $D_2$ receptors and may be important sites for antipsychotic drug action?

A. Locus coeruleus.
B. Caudate and putamen.
C. Raphe nuclei.
D. Nucleus basalis.
E. None of the above.

**The correct response is option B: Caudate and putamen.**

The basal ganglia are relevant to psychiatry because of their chemical anatomy. The caudate and putamen contain a very high concentration of dopamine receptors (option B), particularly $D_2$ receptors. The efficacy of antipsychotic medications is highly correlated with their ability to block $D_2$ receptors. Because $D_2$ receptors have a very high density in these regions, the caudate and putamen may be important sites for antipsychotic drug action. The norepinephrine system arises in the locus coeruleus (option A), whereas the serotonin system arises in the raphe nuclei (option C). The cholinergic system arises in the nucleus basalis (option D). **(pp. 59–61)**

3.3 Which part of the brain is dedicated to speech production?

A. Broca's area.
B. Nucleus basalis.
C. Angular gyrus.
D. Wernicke's area.
E. Amygdala.

**The correct response is option A: Broca's area.**

The left hemisphere contains two major language regions and some subsidiary ones. Broca's area is the region dedicated to the production of speech (option A). It contains information about the syntactical structure of language, provides the "little words" such as prepositions that tie the fabric of language together, and is the generator for fluent speech. Lesions to Broca's area, which occur in stroke victims, lead to halting, stammering, and ungrammatical speech. Wernicke's area (option D) is often referred to as the "auditory association cortex." It encodes the information that permits us to "understand" the sounds expressed in speech. The perception of sound waves, which encode speech, occurs through transducers in the ear that convert the information to neural signals. The signals are received in the auditory cortex, but the meaning of the specific signals cannot be understood (i.e., perceived as constituting words with specific meanings—as opposed, for example, to the wordless music of a symphony) without being compared with "templates" in Wernicke's area. The angular gyrus is a visual association cortex that contains the information or templates that permit us to recognize language presented in visual form (option C). The nucleus basalis (option B) lies in the ventral and medial regions of the globus pallidus and helps mediate memory. The amygdala (option E) forms part of the limbic system and is implicated in a variety of anxiety disorders. **(pp. 62–64)**

3.4   The nucleus accumbens is a key part of which functional system in the brain?

A. Prefrontal system.
B. Limbic system.
C. Memory system.
D. Attention system.
E. Reward system.

**The correct response is option E: Reward system.**

The nucleus accumbens is a key part of the reward system of the brain (option E). Other areas involved in reward processing are the ventral tegmental area, the prefrontal cortex, the amygdala, and the hippocampus. The reward system is relevant to many types of psychiatric disorders. It is often said that substance abuse develops when exposure to a drug such as cocaine "highjacks the brain reward system" by inducing an intense experience of pleasure that stimulates craving and repeated drug-seeking behavior. This system has been implicated in all types of dependence on both illegal (e.g., amphetamines, opiates) and legal (e.g., nicotine, alcohol) substances. It is also thought to provide the basis for other types of pleasure-seeking or addictive behaviors and their consequences, such as gambling disorder or compulsive overeating. **(pp. 64–65)**

3.5 What is the primary neurotransmitter in the brain reward system, which is also associated with adventuresome and exploratory behaviors?

A. Dopamine.
B. Norepinephrine.
C. γ-Aminobutyric acid (GABA).
D. Serotonin.
E. Glutamate.

**The correct response is option A: Dopamine.**

Dopamine is the primary neurotransmitter in the brain reward system and is associated with adventuresome and exploratory behavior (option A). Serotonin (option D) plays a role in modulating mood, anxiety, and aggressive behavior. Norepinephrine (option B) is thought to play a role in mood disorders. Glutamate (option E) is an excitatory neurotransmitter that plays a role in learning and memory. GABA (option C) is of interest because $GABA_A$ receptors contain the binding sites for alcohol, anticonvulsants, and benzodiazepines. Many of the anxiolytic drugs (e.g., the benzodiazepines) act as GABA agonists, thereby increasing the inhibitory tone within the central nervous system. **(pp. 65–71)**

3.6 Where does the brain's noradrenergic system originate?

A. Raphe nuclei.
B. Hypothalamus.
C. Ventral tegmental area.
D. Locus coeruleus.
E. Nucleus accumbens.

**The correct response is option D: Locus coeruleus.**

The noradrenergic system arises in the locus coeruleus and adjacent nuclei that send projections diffusely throughout the entire brain (option D). The serotonin system originates in the raphe nuclei (option A), and the ventral tegmental area (option C) gives rise to the dopamine system. The nucleus accumbens (option E) is important in the reward system. The hypothalamus (option B) receives projections from the locus coeruleus and raphe nuclei, but it is not the site of origin of the noradrenergic or serotonin systems. **(pp. 65–71)**

3.7　Which of the following nuclei in the brain contain the cell bodies of an important group of acetylcholine neurons?

A. Nucleus basalis.
B. Locus coeruleus.
C. Raphe nuclei.
D. Substantia nigra.
E. Caudate nucleus.

**The correct response is option A: Nucleus basalis.**

The nucleus basalis contains the cell bodies of an important group of cholinergic neurons (option A). The locus coeruleus (option B) gives rise to the norepinephrine system, and the raphe nuclei (option C) give rise to the serotonin system. The substantia nigra (option D) contains dopaminergic neurons that have some projections to the caudate nucleus (option E). **(pp. 68–69)**

3.8　Which neurotransmitter regulates arousal, wakefulness, and appetite?

A. Histamine.
B. Acetylcholine.
C. Dopamine.
D. Orexin.
E. Glutamate.

**The correct response is option D: Orexin.**

Orexin regulates arousal, wakefulness, and appetite (option D). Histamine (option A) helps to mediate attention, arousal, and allergic responses. Acetylcholine (option B) plays a major role in the encoding of memory. Glutamate (option E) is an excitatory neurotransmitter. N-methyl-D-aspartate (NMDA) receptors are a part of the glutamate system and help to regulate learning, memory, and the psychotomimetic effects of certain drugs such as phencyclidine. **(pp. 68, 70–71)**

3.9 Family studies of mental illness have shown that most major mental illnesses "run in families." Which of the following is *not* an essential element of a family study?

A. Identifying people with the disorder of interest (e.g., schizophrenia).
B. Identifying people who can serve as control subjects.
C. Interviewing first-degree relatives of ill persons and control subjects.
D. Comparing rates of the disorder of interest in relatives of those with the mental illness in question and relatives of control subjects.
E. Showing that the illness has a definitive genetic component.

**The correct response is option E: Showing that the illness has a definitive genetic component.**

Family studies examine the pattern of aggregation within a family, beginning with the identification of a proband (or index case) who has a disorder of interest, such as bipolar disorder or schizophrenia (option A). Thereafter, all available first-degree relatives (parents, siblings, children) are also evaluated using structured interviews and diagnostic criteria (option C). The prevalence of the specific disorder under investigation is compared with the prevalence in a carefully selected control group (option B). If an increased rate of the specific mental illness under study is observed in the first-degree relatives of the probands as compared with the first-degree relatives of the control subjects, then these results suggest that a disorder is familial and possibly genetic (option D). These studies cannot exclude the possibility that the disorder has prominent nongenetic causes and therefore cannot determine if a disorder has a genetic component (option E). Disorders can also run in families because of learned behavior, role modeling, or predisposing social environments. **(pp. 72–73)**

3.10 Which type of study applies statistical analyses to large databases containing DNA from thousands of individuals affected by specific disorders?

A. Linkage study.
B. Candidate gene study.

C. Genome-wide association study (GWAS).
D. Copy number variant survey.
E. Microarray analysis.

**The correct response is option C: Genome-wide association study (GWAS).**

GWASs apply statistical analyses to large databases containing DNA from thousands of individuals affected by specific disorders (option C). Linkage studies attempt to correlate diseases with specific sites on chromosomes (option A). Candidate gene studies typically begin with hypothesis-driven selection of a candidate gene (option B)—for example, genes encoding neurotransmitter receptors and enzymes such as catechol-*O*-methyltransferase. Microarray analysis is a technique used in molecular biology but is not discussed (option E). Copy number variants, which are mutations in DNA, have the potential to confer disease liability, but a copy number variant survey is not a type of genetic research study (option D). **(p. 74)**

3.11    Which of the following statements accurately characterizes DNA methylation?

A. DNA methylation alters the genome. Methyl groups are added to segments of DNA, turning genes on.
B. DNA methylation alters the genome. Methyl groups are added to segments of DNA, turning genes off.
C. DNA methylation does not alter the genome. Methyl groups are added to segments of DNA, turning genes on.
D. DNA methylation does not alter the genome. Methyl groups are added to segments of DNA, turning genes off.
E. None of the above.

**The correct response is option D: DNA methylation does not alter the genome. Methyl groups are added to segments of DNA, turning genes off.**

DNA methylation is an epigenetic process. Epigenetic processes turn genes off or on *without* altering the genome (options A and B). DNA methylation turns genes off (option D) rather than on (option C). **(p. 75)**

# — CHAPTER 4 —

# Neurodevelopmental (Child) Disorders

4.1    What is the standard test used to assess the intelligence of children between ages 6 and 16 years?

A. Stanford-Binet Intelligence Scale.
B. Wechsler Intelligence Scale for Children—Fifth Edition (WISC-V).
C. Weschler Individual Achievement Test.
D. Kaufman Assessment Battery for Children.
E. Wechsler Preschool and Primary Scale of Intelligence.

**The correct response is option B: Wechsler Intelligence Scale for Children—Fifth Edition (WISC-V).**

The WISC-V is the standard instrument for assessing the intelligence of school-age children between ages 6 and 16 years (option B). Younger children can be assessed with the Kaufman Assessment Battery for Children (option D) or the Wechsler Preschool and Primary Scale of Intelligence (option E). The WISC-V consists of a group of 10 core subtests that assess a variety of cognitive functions (e.g., vocabulary, comprehension, block design, matrix reasoning, digit span, symbol search). These are used to generate a full-scale IQ, verbal and performance IQs, and four composite scores known as indices (verbal comprehension, perceptual organization, processing speed, and working memory). The Stanford-Binet Intelligence Scale (option A) is one of the oldest scales and can be used for some younger children. The Weschler Individual Achievement Test (option C) measures listening, speaking, reading, writing, and mathematical skills in individuals ages 4–50 years. Evaluating the pattern of achievement can provide some index as to whether the child has a learning disorder. **(pp. 86–87)**

4.2    Intellectual disabilities are characterized by which of the following?

A. IQ measured to be at least two standard deviations below the mean and deficits in adaptive functioning.
B. Deficits in intellectual functions without regard to adaptive functioning.
C. Deficits in intellectual functions and deficits in adaptive functioning.
D. Deficits in adaptive functioning without regard to intellectual functions.
E. IQ measured to be at least three standard deviations below the mean regardless of deficits in adaptive functioning.

**The correct response is option C: Deficits in intellectual functions and deficits in adaptive functioning.**

A diagnosis of intellectual disability requires evidence of intellectual disability confirmed by both clinical assessment and standardized intelligence testing (option C), unlike DSM-IV's mental retardation, which had been defined exclusively on the basis of IQ. Because IQ is not part of the definition of intellectual disability, options A and E are incorrect. Options B and D are incorrect because the diagnosis requires *both* intellectual deficits and deficits in adaptive functioning. **(pp. 87–90)**

4.3    What is the most common heritable cause of intellectual disability?

A. Down syndrome.
B. Fragile X syndrome.
C. Tay-Sachs disease.
D. Prader-Willi syndrome.
E. Williams syndrome.

**The correct response is option B: Fragile X syndrome.**

Fragile X syndrome is the most common heritable cause of intellectual disability (option B). Down syndrome is the most common chromosomal cause (option A). Options C–E are less common causes of intellectual disability. **(pp. 90–91)**

4.4    A 25-year-old man with intellectual disability has lived in a group home throughout his adult life. He can read his name and a few other words. He can take care of his activities of daily living such as bathing and other personal hygiene tasks and doing laundry. He was in special education classes throughout school. What is the probable severity of his intellectual disability?

A. Mild.
B. Moderate.
C. Severe.
D. Profound.
E. Unable to estimate.

**The correct response is option B: Moderate.**

This patient's level of impairment is consistent with moderate intellectual disability (option B). Patients with mild intellectual disability (option A) are capable of living in the community, working, reading, writing, and doing basic arithmetic. Patients with severe and profound intellectual disability (options C, D) generally require an institutionalized care setting. **(pp. 89–90)**

4.5    A mother of an 8-year-old girl asks her family doctor what she can do about her child's speech impediment. The girl displays frequent repetitions or prolongations of sounds, often pauses in the middle of a word, and frequently fills her speech with "um" or "like," which she then repeats ("um-um-um"). Which of the following is the girl's most likely communication disorder?

A. Language disorder.
B. Speech sound disorder.
C. Childhood-onset fluency disorder.
D. Social (pragmatic) communication disorder.
E. Autism spectrum disorder.

**The correct response is option C: Childhood-onset fluency disorder.**

The child displays stuttering, and childhood-onset fluency disorder is the correct diagnosis (option C). Language disorder (option A) is a deficit in comprehension or production of language. Speech sound disorder (option B) is a disorder of speech production that accounts for phenomena such as articulation errors. Children who have difficulty tailoring their communication appropriately to the social context are diagnosed with social (pragmatic) communication disorder (option D). Patients with autism spectrum disorder (option E) have difficulties with social communication and display a pattern of restricted, stereotyped interests. **(pp. 92–93)**

4.6     An 8-year-old boy is brought to a child psychiatrist for an evaluation. His parents report that he is socially awkward and has trouble making friends, but his grades have always been good. The boy is polite but overly formal in conversation. He avoids eye contact. His parents report that he sticks to a rigid routine at home and has an unusually intense interest in U.S. presidents and can name all of them in correct order. When this topic is brought up, the boy begins a lengthy discourse on them. Which of the following is the best diagnosis?

A. Language disorder.
B. Speech sound disorder.
C. Childhood-onset fluency disorder.
D. Social (pragmatic) communication disorder.
E. Autism spectrum disorder.

**The correct response is option E: Autism spectrum disorder.**

Patients with autism spectrum disorder have difficulties with social communication and display a pattern of restricted, stereotyped interests (option E). Language disorder (option A) is a deficit in comprehension or production of language. Speech sound disorder (option B) is a disorder of speech production that accounts for phenomena such as articulation errors. Social (pragmatic) communication disorder (option D) is a diagnosis used in children who have difficulty tailoring their communication appropriately to the social context but do not have the pattern of restricted, stereotyped interests seen in autism spectrum disorder. Childhood-onset fluency disorder (option C) is a diagnosis for children who stutter. **(pp. 92–98)**

4.7    Treatment with stimulant medications in children with attention-deficit/hyperactivity disorder (ADHD)...

A. Increases risk for later substance abuse.
B. Decreases risk for later substance abuse.
C. Does not affect risk for substance abuse.
D. Is associated with a worse long-term outcome of ADHD.
E. Increases risk for abuse of stimulant medications only.

**The correct response is option B: Decreases risk for later substance abuse.**

Research shows that using stimulant medications to treat ADHD decreases the patient's risk for later substance abuse (option B). Treating ADHD brings symptomatic relief and can lead to a better long-term outcome. **(p. 104)**

4.8    What is the prevalence of ADHD in children?

A. 1%–2%.
B. 5%.
C. 10%.
D. 20%.
E. >30%.

**The correct response is option B: 5%.**

The prevalence of ADHD in children is about 5% (option B), and for that reason options A, C, D, and E are incorrect. **(p. 103)**

4.9    A 9-year-old boy is brought to his pediatrician by his parents, who are concerned about the possibility of ADHD. His teacher says that he is frequently in trouble for fighting with other children and that he refuses to obey classroom rules. He frequently steals small items from his peers and the school cafeteria. He also talks out of turn and has trouble staying in his seat. His parents report that he has lots of energy and that he "bounces off the walls" at home. He talks back to his parents. Which of the following symptoms in this case is most suggestive of ADHD?

A. Fighting with other children.
B. Refusal to obey classroom rules.

C. Stealing.

D. Talking back to parents.

E. Difficulty staying in his seat.

**The correct response is option E: Difficulty staying in his seat.**

Having trouble staying seated is typical of children with ADHD (option E). Fighting and stealing (options A, C) suggest a diagnosis of conduct disorder, symptoms that are not included in the definition of ADHD. Refusing to obey rules and talking back to parents (options B, D) are suggestive of either conduct disorder or oppositional defiant disorder rather than ADHD. All these disorders can co-occur, however. **(pp. 99–101)**

4.10 The pediatrician caring for the boy described in the previous vignette (4.9) has decided to prescribe medication to target ADHD. Which of the following response options is considered a first-line treatment?

A. Guanfacine.

B. Methylphenidate.

C. Clonidine.

D. Risperidone.

E. Atomoxetine.

**The correct response is option B: Methylphenidate.**

Methylphenidate is one of the first-line treatments for ADHD (option B), the other being amphetamine salts. Atomoxetine (option E), guanfacine (option A), and clonidine (option C) are second-line treatments. Risperidone (option D) is incorrect because it is a second-generation antipsychotic U.S. Food and Drug Administration (FDA)–approved to treat irritability in children with autism spectrum disorder. **(pp. 99, 105)**

4.11 Which of the following is *not* a common side effect of the stimulant medications commonly used to treat ADHD?

A. Weight gain.

B. Insomnia.

C. Stomach upset.

D. Irritability.

E. Appetite suppression.

**The correct response is option A: Weight gain.**

Weight loss, not weight gain (option A), is a common side effect of stimulants. For this reason, weight should be monitored in children prescribed stimulants. Options B–E are common side effects of stimulants. **(p. 105)**

4.12 A 9-year-old boy of average intelligence is making satisfactory grades in all subjects in school except math, which he is failing. His Iowa Test of Basic Skills score confirms satisfactory performance on all subjects except math, which is considerably lower than average. He sometimes shows irritation and frustration in the classroom during math class, but his behavior is otherwise unremarkable. His parents do not have concerns about his mood or behavior at home. Which of the following response options will be most beneficial for this child?

A. Remedial instruction in math and instruction in compensatory learning strategies.

B. Methylphenidate.

C. Fluoxetine.

D. Atomoxetine.

E. Cognitive-behavioral therapy.

**The correct response is option A: Remedial instruction in math and instruction in compensatory learning strategies.**

This boy has a specific learning disorder, which is an inability to achieve in a designated area of learning at a level consistent with the person's overall intellectual functioning. Specific learning disorders are common and affect 5%–15% of school-age children and are more common in boys. The usual treatment for a specific learning disorder is remedial instruction in the area of weakness (option A) plus learning compensatory strategies. Medications and cognitive-behavioral therapy (options B–E) have no role in its treatment. **(pp. 106–107)**

4.13   Which of the following response options is *not* considered a stereotypic movement when considering the diagnosis of stereotypic movement disorder?

A. Head banging.
B. Rocking.
C. Hitting one's own body.
D. Nonrhythmic, jerky movements of the neck.
E. Hand waving.

**The correct response is option D: Nonrhythmic, jerky movements of the neck.**

Stereotypic movement disorder is characterized by repetitive, often seemingly driven, and apparently purposeless motor behaviors that interfere with social, academic, and other activities or result in self-injury. Nonrhythmic, jerky movements of the neck (option D) are better classified as tics. Options A–C and E can be types of stereotypic movements. **(p. 108)**

4.14   How does the diagnosis of Tourette's disorder differ from a persistent motor or vocal tic disorder?

A. Patients with Tourette's disorder have coprolalia (offensive vocal tics).
B. Tics in Tourette's disorder are of longer duration than tics that occur in motor or vocal tic disorder.
C. Patients with Tourette's disorder have both motor and vocal tics.
D. Tourette's disorder is associated with streptococcal infection.
E. Tourette's disorder has high comorbidity with obsessive-compulsive disorder.

**The correct response is option C: Patients with Tourette's disorder have both motor and vocal tics.**

Patients with Tourette's disorder have both motor and vocal tics, which differentiates this disorder from chronic motor or vocal tic disorder (option C), in which the patients have only motor or vocal tics but not both. The vocal tics accompanying Tourette's disorder can be somewhat socially offensive (option A). Tics tend to be of similar duration regardless of specific diagnosis (option B).

Some cases of Tourette's disorder are associated with streptococ-cal infection (option D) and may have comorbidity with obses-sive-compulsive disorder (option E), but these features do not need to be present for diagnosis. **(pp. 108–110)**

4.15   Which of the following medications are FDA approved to treat pediatric depression?

A. Fluoxetine and escitalopram.
B. Citalopram and paroxetine.
C. Venlafaxine and nefazodone.
D. Sertraline and citalopram.
E. Escitalopram and citalopram.

**The correct response is option A: Fluoxetine and escitalopram.**

Mood disorders are common in children and adolescents. Up to 5% of children and 8% of adolescents meet diagnostic criteria for major depression. A combination of medication and psychother-apy is usually recommended to provide the best chance for re-covery. Fluoxetine and escitalopram are FDA approved for the treatment of pediatric depression (option A) and should be used as first-line medications. The antidepressants listed in response options B–E are not approved to treat pediatric depression. **(p. 111)**

# — CHAPTER 5 —

# Schizophrenia Spectrum and Other Psychotic Disorders

5.1   Which of the following statements *mischaracterizes* schizophrenia?

A. Patients have a "split" personality.
B. Patients have disability in their capacity to think clearly.
C. Patients have disability in their capacity to experience normal emotions.
D. Patients typically develop symptoms in early adulthood.
E. Patients often develop bizarre hallucinations and delusions.

**The correct response is option A: Patients have a "split" personality.**

Patients with schizophrenia do not have a split personality (option A) or multiple personalities. Options B–E are generally true of schizophrenia. **(pp. 115, 124–129)**

5.2   A 45-year-old man has sought help for "stress." He attributes his stress to what he believes is a conspiracy by coworkers to get him fired by "arranging" work-related incidents that reflect poorly on him, such as hiding reports he's written or stealing needed documents. He has threatened to sue the coworkers, who have denied the allegations. As his psychiatrist, you find yourself unable to get him to talk about other issues. He has no auditory or visual hallucinations or any history of a mood disorder. His dress

and grooming are appropriate, and his thoughts are well organized. Which of the following is the most likely diagnosis?

A. Schizophrenia.
B. Schizoaffective disorder.
C. Schizophreniform disorder.
D. Delusional disorder.
E. Bipolar I disorder.

**The correct response is option D: Delusional disorder.**

People with a delusional disorder have delusions accompanied
by minimal (or no) hallucinations, and their behavior apart from
the delusion or its ramifications is not markedly bizarre or odd
(option D). These individuals are often described as overtalk-
ative and circumstantial, particularly when discussing their delusions. They do not exhibit other symptoms of schizophrenia
(option A) and schizophreniform disorder (option C) such as disorganized thinking or behavior. Schizoaffective disorder (option
B) and bipolar I disorder (option E) are not likely given the absence of a mood disturbance. **(pp. 116–121)**

5.3    At what age do women typically develop schizophrenia?

A. 13–18 years.
B. 18–25 years.
C. 21–30 years.
D. 35–50 years.
E. >50 years.

**The correct response is option C: 21–30 years.**

Women typically develop symptoms between ages 21 and 30 years
(option C). Men typically develop symptoms between ages 18
and 25. **(p. 124)**

5.4    Which of the following is an example of a "first-rank" symptom
of schizophrenia as identified by psychiatrist Kurt Schneider?

A. The patient believes that thoughts are being inserted into his
or her mind.
B. The patient believes that the government is spying on him or her.

C. The patient believes that his or her masturbation has led to insanity.
D. The patient believes the somatic delusion that his or her heart has stopped beating.
E. The patient experiences the tactile hallucination that insects are crawling under his or her skin.

**The correct response is option A: The patient believes that thoughts are being inserted into his or her mind.**

Schneider, a German psychiatrist working in the early twentieth century, argued that certain types of hallucinations and delusions were of the "first rank," meaning that they are especially characteristic of schizophrenia. Examples include delusions of being forced to do things against one's will or that thoughts are being withdrawn from or inserted into one's mind (option A). These symptoms all reflect a patient's confusion about the loss of boundaries between himself or herself and the external world. Options B–D are examples of delusions commonly seen in persons with psychosis but are not examples of "first-rank" delusions. Option E refers to *formication*, which is a hallucination in which the person feels that insects are crawling under his or her skin and is also not considered a first-rank symptom. **(p. 126)**

5.5    You are evaluating a 30-year-old woman with schizophrenia admitted to a psychiatric inpatient unit. She believes that she is dead and no longer exists. She will not accept any evidence to the contrary. What type of delusion is this?

A. Persecutory delusion.
B. Grandiose delusion.
C. Nihilistic delusion.
D. Somatic delusion.
E. Religious delusion.

**The correct response is option C: Nihilistic delusion.**

Patients with nihilistic delusions believe that they are dead or dying (option C) or that they or the world does not exist. Grandiose delusions (option B) involve the patient having special powers or eminence. Persecutory delusions (option A) have as their theme being spied on or plotted against. Somatic delusions (option D) involve bodily functions ("my heart has stopped beating"). Religious delusions (option E) tend to concern having a special relationship with a higher power or a special religious mission. **(Table 5–2 [Varied content in delusions], p. 125)**

5.6 Which phase of schizophrenia is characterized by subtle behavior changes that include social withdrawal, work impairment, blunting of emotion, avolition, and odd ideas and behavior?

A. Prodromal phase.
B. Active phase.
C. Residual phase.
D. Cataleptic phase.
E. Schizoaffective phase.

**The correct response is option A: Prodromal phase.**

The prodromal phase of schizophrenia is characterized by subtle behavior changes that include social withdrawal, work impairment, blunting of emotion, avolition, and odd ideas and behavior (option A). This phase precedes the active phase (option B), in which full-blown psychotic symptoms occur, such as hallucinations, delusions, or disorganized speech and behavior. The residual phase is characterized by role impairment, negative symptoms, and attenuated positive symptoms (option C). The terms *cataleptic* and *schizoaffective* (options D, E) do not refer to typical phases of schizophrenia. **(Table 5–4 [Typical stages of schizophrenia], p. 130)**

5.7 You are treating a patient with schizophrenia on a psychiatric inpatient unit. The patient has displayed disorganized thinking and behavior throughout hospitalization, such as tangential speech and dressing in a bizarre manner. One day at morning rounds, the patient mimics your hand gestures without explanation. What is the term for this behavior?

A. Echolalia.
B. Echopraxia.
C. Catatonic stupor.
D. Negativism.
E. Stereotypy.

**The correct response is option B: Echopraxia.**

Echopraxia is a type of disorganized behavior in which a patient will mimic an examiner's movements or mannerisms (option B). Echolalia is manifested when a patient repeats things said in his or her presence (option A). Catatonic stupor is when a patient is immobile, mute, and unresponsive, yet fully conscious (option C). Negativism occurs when a patient refuses to perform simple requests for no apparent reason (option D). A stereotypy (option E) is a purposeless repetitive movement, such as rocking back and forth. **(pp. 127, 156)**

5.8     A 20-year-old man with schizophrenia comes to your clinic for a scheduled follow-up visit, accompanied by his mother, with whom he lives. His disorder is well controlled with a second-generation antipsychotic. He reports mild auditory hallucinations but is not bothered by them. His mother is concerned that her son is inactive much of the day and must be prompted to groom himself. He prefers to watch TV all day without engaging in any other activities. The patient shows some affective blunting but has not had depressive or manic symptoms during his illness. He reports restful sleep and has a healthy appetite. He tolerates his medication without noticeable adverse effects and says he feels "pretty good" about his current situation. How should you address the mother's concerns?

A. Prescribe a stimulant to increase his energy.
B. Prescribe an antidepressant to treat his negative symptoms.
C. Reassess the patient for schizoaffective disorder and consider adding a mood stabilizer.
D. Reduce the dose of the antipsychotic.
E. Provide psychoeducation to the patient's mother.

**The correct response is option E: Provide psychoeducation to the patient's mother.**

Avolition—lack of initiative or goals—is a common negative symptom of schizophrenia with no effective medical treatments. As such, it is wise to educate the family about schizophrenia and its many symptoms (option E), including avolition. Stimulants could lead to a worsening of the patient's psychosis (option A). Antidepressants are not clearly indicated because the patient has no depressive symptoms (option B). Reducing the dose of the antipsychotic medication (option D) could lead to relapse of positive symptoms, and it is not clear that this would help the patient with his negative symptoms. Furthermore, he is taking a low dose of an antipsychotic and does not report adverse effects. The patient has not had a clear-cut depressive or manic episode, so there is no reason to diagnose schizoaffective disorder (option C). **(pp. 134–140)**

5.9  A 24-year-old woman is admitted to an inpatient psychiatric unit for acute psychosis. She endorses auditory hallucinations and persecutory delusions and has an inappropriate affect. She has had no previous episodes and has not abused substances, and a medical workup is negative. She has not had symptoms of depression or mania. At this point, her total duration of illness is 2 weeks. Which of the following is the best diagnosis?

A. Schizophrenia.
B. Schizoaffective disorder.
C. Schizophreniform disorder.
D. Brief psychotic disorder.
E. Bipolar disorder.

**The correct response is option D: Brief psychotic disorder.**

Because the total duration of illness is less than 1 month, the appropriate diagnosis is brief psychotic disorder (option D). Patients with a total duration of illness from 1 month to 6 months should be diagnosed with schizophreniform disorder (option C). Patients whose total duration of illness exceeds 6 months should be diagnosed with schizophrenia (option A). Schizoaffective disorder (option B) and bipolar disorder (option E) are not appropriate diagnoses because there is no evidence of a mood disturbance. **(pp. 121–122)**

5.10  Peripartum onset is a specifier for which DSM-5 psychotic disorder?

A. Schizophrenia.
B. Schizoaffective disorder.
C. Schizophreniform disorder.
D. Brief psychotic disorder.
E. Bipolar disorder.

**The correct response is option D: Brief psychotic disorder.**

According to DSM-5, peripartum onset is a specifier of brief psychotic disorder (option D), and it should be coded as brief psychotic disorder with peripartum onset. Peripartum onset is not a specifier of options A–C or E. **(p. 121)**

5.11 A 24-year-old woman is admitted to an inpatient psychiatric unit after developing a recurrence of psychotic symptoms in the setting of medication noncompliance. She hears voices telling her not to take her medication and thinks her psychiatrist is poisoning her. For that reason, she stopped taking her antipsychotic 2 weeks earlier. She denies abusing substances, and a urine drug screen is negative. There are no clear symptoms of depression or of mania. Two months earlier, she experienced her first psychotic episode, which lasted for 3 weeks but resolved with antipsychotic medication. Which of the following is the best diagnosis?

A. Schizophrenia.
B. Schizoaffective disorder.
C. Schizophreniform disorder.
D. Brief psychotic disorder.
E. Bipolar disorder.

**The correct response is option C: Schizophreniform disorder.**

The schizophreniform disorder diagnosis is used with patients who have psychotic symptoms suggestive of schizophrenia but whose total duration of illness falls between 1 month and 6 months (option C). Brief psychotic disorder (option D) has a maximum duration of 1 month, and the diagnosis of schizophrenia (option A) is reserved for patients whose total duration of illness exceeds 6 months. Schizoaffective disorder (option B) and bipolar disorder (option E) are not appropriate diagnoses in the absence of mood symptoms. **(p. 122)**

5.12 Which of the following risk factors is associated with poor outcome in schizophrenia?

A. Female gender.
B. Insidious onset of symptoms.
C. Short prodrome.

D. Married or partnered.

E. Later onset.

**The correct response is option B: Insidious onset of symptoms.**

Insidious onset of symptoms in schizophrenia is associated with poor outcome (option B). Options A and C–E are all associated with better outcomes. **(Table 5–5 [Features associated with good and poor outcome in schizophrenia], p. 131)**

5.13 Which of the following brain abnormalities in schizophrenia is associated with poor premorbid functioning, negative symptoms, poor response to treatment, and cognitive impairment?

A. Sulcal enlargement.

B. Cerebellar atrophy.

C. Decreased size of frontal lobe.

D. Ventricular enlargement.

E. Decreased size of thalamus.

**The correct response is option D: Ventricular enlargement.**

Ventricular enlargement in schizophrenia is associated with poor premorbid functioning, negative symptoms, poor response to treatment, and cognitive impairment (option D). Options A–C and E reflect other brain abnormalities that have been associated with schizophrenia but have not been specifically tied to poor outcome or negative symptoms. **(pp. 132–133)**

5.14 Which of the following individuals has the lowest risk for developing schizophrenia?

A. Sibling of a person with schizophrenia.

B. Member of the general population.

C. Identical twin of a person with schizophrenia.

D. Nonidentical twin of a person with schizophrenia.

E. Child having one parent with schizophrenia.

**The correct response is option B: Member of the general population.**

Members of the general population have a 0.5%–1% risk for schizophrenia (option B). Siblings of a person with schizophrenia carry a 10% risk for schizophrenia (option A). Identical twins of a person with schizophrenia carry a 46% risk, whereas nonidentical twins carry a 14% risk (options C, D). Children having one parent with schizophrenia have a 5%–6% risk for schizophrenia (option E). **(pp. 124, 132)**

5.15   A 30-year-old woman with auditory hallucinations and persecutory delusions is admitted to an inpatient psychiatric unit after developing euphoria, insomnia, agitation, and pressured speech. Her psychotic symptoms are usually well controlled with risperidone, a second-generation antipsychotic. She has a history of major depressive episodes, but she has psychotic symptoms even after the episodes resolve. What is the usual treatment for her disorder?

A. Switch to clozapine from risperidone.
B. Add lithium or valproate to the risperidone.
C. Start a selective serotonin reuptake inhibitor (SSRI) antidepressant.
D. Add the first-generation antipsychotic haloperidol to the risperidone.
E. Add the benzodiazepine clonazepam to the risperidone.

**The correct response is option B: Add lithium or valproate to the risperidone.**

The patient in this vignette has schizoaffective disorder, bipolar type. This is indicated by her manic syndrome, history of major depression, and ongoing psychotic symptoms. Because the patient is manic, the best next step is to add a mood stabilizer, such as lithium or valproate (option B). Clozapine (option A) could be an option in cases of treatment-refractory schizophrenia but is a second-line choice because of agranulocytosis risk. Its use in treating schizoaffective disorder is "off-label." Starting an antidepressant (option C) would be helpful for a patient with schizoaffective disorder with an acute depressive episode but is not applicable here. Adding a second antipsychotic (option D) should not be considered before a trial of a mood stabilizer. Adding a benzodiazepine (option E) might be helpful for acute agitation, but it would not be a primary treatment for schizoaffective disorder, bipolar type. **(pp. 137–140)**

5.16  Which of the following mechanisms of action has been hypothe-
      sized to explain the effectiveness of antipsychotic medications?

      A. Dopamine ($D_2$) receptor blockade.
      B. 5-Hydroxytryptamine (serotonin) type 2 receptor (5-HT$_2$)
         blockade.
      C. Glutamate receptor blockade.
      D. Inhibition of serotonin reuptake.
      E. Inhibition of dopamine reuptake.

**The correct response is option A: Dopamine ($D_2$) receptor
blockade.**

The main mechanism of action of antipsychotics is thought to be
their ability to block $D_2$ receptors (option A). Second-generation
antipsychotics also block 5-HT$_2$ receptors (option B). Glutamate
is thought to play a role in schizophrenia, but agents that affect
glutamatergic neurotransmission have no current role in the
treatment of schizophrenia (option C). Options D and E play an
important role for several medications but are not discussed in
this chapter and are not plausible responses. **(pp. 133–134)**

5.17  Which of the following psychosocial treatments has been shown
      to reduce rates of relapse in schizophrenia?

      A. Cognitive-behavioral therapy.
      B. Interpersonal psychotherapy.
      C. Social skills training.
      D. Family therapy.
      E. Vocational rehabilitation.

**The correct response is option D: Family therapy.**

Family therapy, combined with antipsychotic medication, has been
shown to reduce relapse rates in schizophrenia (option D). Families need realistic and accurate information about the symptoms,
course of illness, and available treatments. They also will benefit
from learning how to improve communications with their
schizophrenic relative and how to provide constructive support.
Although options A–C and E may have value, their effectiveness
in reducing relapse rates is not established. **(pp. 135–136)**

5.18    Which of the following response options is consistent with a di-
        agnosis of schizoaffective disorder but not major depression or
        bipolar disorder?

        A. Manic episodes accompanied by hallucinations and delu-
           sions.
        B. Depressive episodes accompanied by hallucinations and de-
           lusions.
        C. Hallucinations and delusions for at least 2 weeks in the ab-
           sence of a major mood episode.
        D. Presence of a mixed mood episode accompanied by halluci-
           nations and delusions.
        E. Symptoms of a major mood episode present for 25% of the to-
           tal duration of the illness.

        **The correct response is option C: Hallucinations and delusions
        for at least 2 weeks in the absence of a major mood episode.**

        The hallmark of schizoaffective disorder is the presence of either
        a depressive or a manic episode concurrent with symptoms char-
        acteristic of schizophrenia, such as delusions, hallucinations, or
        disorganized speech. Hallucinations or delusions must be pres-
        ent for 2 weeks or more in the absence of prominent mood symp-
        toms (option C), but mood symptoms must be present for most
        of the total duration of the illness (option E). If the total duration
        of the mood episodes is less than 50% of the total duration of the
        illness, schizophrenia is the likely diagnosis. Options A, B, and D
        are consistent with a diagnosis of a psychotic mood disorder.
        **(pp. 137–140)**

# — CHAPTER 6 —

# Mood Disorders

6.1    Who first differentiated bipolar disorder from schizophrenia?

A. Eugen Bleuler.
B. Emil Kraepelin.
C. Sigmund Freud.
D. Kurt Schneider.
E. Carl Jung.

**The correct response is option B: Emil Kraepelin.**

Kraepelin differentiated bipolar disorder from schizophrenia (option B), although the terms he used at the time were *manic-depressive insanity* and *dementia praecox*, respectively. Bleuler (option A) coined the term *schizophrenia*. Schneider (option D) is noted for identifying "first-rank" symptoms thought to be pathognomonic for schizophrenia. Freud and Jung (options C, E) were famous psychoanalysts who made important contributions to psychiatry but who had no role in separating bipolar disorder from schizophrenia. **(pp. 126–127, 141–142)**

6.2    What is the minimum duration of a manic episode?

A. 12 hours.
B. 1–2 days.
C. 4 days.
D. 7 days.
E. 2 weeks.

**The correct response is option D: 7 days.**

A manic episode must last at least 7 days according to DSM-5 (option D). A hypomanic episode must last at least 4 days. A major depressive episode must last at least 2 weeks. In the case of mood reactivity lasting from hours up to a day or two, consider affective instability associated with a personality disorder such as borderline personality disorder or cyclothymia. **(pp. 142–143)**

6.3    Which of the following features is consistent with a hypomanic episode but *not* a manic episode?

A. Presence of hallucinations and delusions.
B. Duration of at least 1 week.
C. Elevated mood.
D. Decreased need for sleep.
E. Lack of marked social and occupational dysfunction.

**The correct response is option E: Lack of marked social and occupational dysfunction.**

Hypomanic episodes are different from manic episodes because they do not cause as much social or occupational dysfunction (option E), nor do they typically result in psychiatric hospitalization. Hypomanic episodes are not associated with psychotic symptoms, but psychotic symptoms can occur in manic episodes (option A). Hypomanic episodes must last at least 4 days, but they do not have a specified maximum duration in DSM-5 (option B). Elevated mood and decreased need for sleep (options C, D) can occur in both manic and hypomanic episodes. **(pp. 142–143, 146)**

6.4    A 28-year-old man is brought to the emergency department by the police for a psychiatric evaluation after his neighbors reported that he was behaving erratically. He is irritable with pressured speech and has slept only a few hours in the past several days. He believes that the FBI has implanted a microchip in his brain to record his thoughts and send him messages. He has been spending several hours each day making blueprints for lethal booby traps for his home to protect himself against government agents. He derails frequently in conversation. His physical examination is significant for dental caries, and his urine drug screen is positive for amphetamines. Why would it be premature to diagnose this patient with bipolar I disorder based on this presentation?

A. Presence of psychosis.
B. Persecutory delusions.
C. Mood is irritable rather than elevated.
D. Amphetamines present in drug screen.
E. Lack of grandiosity.

**The correct response is option D: Amphetamines present in drug screen.**

Without further information, it is premature to diagnose this patient with bipolar I disorder, because methamphetamine intoxication can induce manic symptoms (option D). Per DSM-5, it must be determined that manic symptoms are not attributable to the physiological effects of a substance. In this case, collateral information about the time course of illness should be obtained, because patients with bipolar disorders are often disinhibited and more likely to use illicit drugs during mania. Options A–C and E do not rule out bipolar I disorder. As a side note, a paranoid psychosis and dental caries ("meth mouth") are suggestive of a methamphetamine use disorder. **(pp. 142–143, 366)**

6.5    A 10-year-old boy is brought to his family physician by his parents. He has had recurrent severe behavioral outbursts at home and at school several times a week for the past several years. Outbursts are typically in reaction to minor disappointments or when he is asked to do routine chores. His parents did not seek attention for this problem because they thought he would outgrow it. Between outbursts, the boy's mood is "grumpy." Which of the following is the most likely diagnosis?

A. Disruptive mood dysregulation disorder.
B. Bipolar II disorder.
C. Major depressive disorder.
D. Persistent depressive disorder.
E. Unspecified depressive disorder.

**The correct response is option A: Disruptive mood dysregulation disorder.**

Disruptive mood dysregulation disorder is new to DSM-5 for children and adolescents with recurrent, severe behavioral outbursts (option A). Prior to DSM-5, many of these children received a diagnosis of bipolar disorder, even though they tended not to develop a typical adult bipolar disorder characterized by recurrent manic and depressive episodes. A disruptive mood dysregulation disorder diagnosis can coexist with other depressive disorders. In this case, it is the primary diagnosis because information provided in the vignette is insufficient to diagnose a comorbid depressive disorder. **(pp. 147–149)**

6.6 A 35-year-old woman comes to your clinic to establish care. She reports that she has been depressed since adolescence with ongoing symptoms of low mood throughout the day, feelings of worthlessness, and low energy. She does not remember any recent period in the past several years that she was free of depression. Which of the following is the best diagnosis?

A. Major depressive disorder.
B. Persistent depressive disorder.
C. Disruptive mood dysregulation disorder.
D. Unspecified depressive disorder.
E. Bipolar II disorder.

**The correct response is option B: Persistent depressive disorder.**

Patients with continuous symptoms of depression for 2 years or more should be diagnosed with persistent depressive disorder (option B). Only two symptoms are required in addition to depressed mood. Because she reports only two symptoms, she does not meet criteria for major depressive disorder (option A). Disruptive mood dysregulation disorder (option C) is a diagnosis for children with severe and persistent irritability. Bipolar II disorder (option E) cannot entirely be ruled out because the vignette is silent on past manic or hypomanic symptoms. Because this patient appears to meet the criteria for persistent depressive disorder, unspecified depressive disorder (option D) is inappropriate because it is a diagnosis of exclusion. **(pp. 154–156)**

6.7 A 30-year-old man comes to your clinic seeking help for depression. He reports feeling depressed most of each day for the past 3 weeks. He complains of poor sleep, low energy, inability to concentrate, and diminished appetite. He has lost interest in his work, and he spends much of his time watching TV. He has lost 5 pounds. He has had thoughts of hanging himself but does not think he would actually try to kill himself because of responsibility to his family. This is his fourth episode of depression since adolescence, and he has no history of mania or hypomania. Previous episodes have resolved spontaneously within a few months, and he is symptom free between episodes. Which of the following is the best diagnosis?

A. Disruptive mood dysregulation disorder.
B. Bipolar I disorder.
C. Major depressive disorder.
D. Persistent depressive disorder.
E. Unspecified depressive disorder.

**The correct response is option C: Major depressive disorder.**

The patient's symptoms meet criteria for major depressive disorder (option C). The patient does not have persistent depressive disorder (option D) because his symptoms are episodic rather than chronic. Persistent depressive disorder also tends to be of milder severity. There is no evidence of a bipolar I disorder because he has no history of mania (option B). Disruptive mood dysregulation disorder (option A) is a diagnosis for persistently irritable children, whereas unspecified depressive disorder (option E) is a diagnosis of exclusion. **(pp. 149–154)**

6.8    A 60-year-old woman develops depressive symptoms following the death of her husband 1 month earlier. She reports trouble sleeping, feelings of guilt, low energy, and decreased appetite. She has difficulty paying attention to conversations with friends. She has thoughts about wanting to go to sleep and not wake up, thereby "joining" her deceased husband. When explored, it turns out that the patient's guilty feelings related to not telling her husband how much he was loved. The patient denies previous episodes of depression. Which of the following is the best diagnosis?

A. Bereavement.
B. Major depressive disorder.
C. Unspecified depressive disorder.

D. Persistent depressive disorder.

E. Bipolar II disorder.

**The correct response is option A: Bereavement.**

Because of the recent death of her husband, and in the absence of previous depressive episodes, the best response is bereavement (option A). Bereavement is typically considered a normal and expected response to significant loss and can lead to feelings of intense sadness, rumination about the loss, insomnia, poor appetite, and weight loss. That said, major depressive disorder (option B) is a credible response, because the line between bereavement and a major depressive episode is slim. The distinction often comes down to the clinician's judgment based on the individual's history and the cultural norms for the patient. The vignette does not provide evidence of mania or hypomania; thus, option E is unlikely. Persistent depressive disorder (option D) is incorrect because the patient's symptoms are episodic rather than chronic. Unspecified depressive disorder is inappropriate because it is a diagnosis of exclusion (option C). **(pp. 149–153)**

6.9    What does it mean for a patient with bipolar disorder to have "rapid-cycling"?

A. Severe mood swings throughout the day.

B. Switching between mania and depression several times throughout a week.

C. At least four distinct mood episodes (e.g., mania, depression) in 1 year.

D. At least four distinct mood episodes (e.g., mania, depression) in 1 month.

E. None of the above.

**The correct response is option C: At least four distinct mood episodes (e.g., mania, depression) in 1 year.**

Rapid-cycling indicates the presence of at least four distinct mood episodes in 1 year (option C). Rapid-cycling bipolar disorder is a particularly severe form of the disorder and is associated with a younger age at onset, more frequent depressive episodes, and greater risk for suicide attempts than other forms of the disorder. **(p. 158)**

6.10 A major depressive episode characterized by interpersonal rejection sensitivity, increased appetite, and hypersomnia indicates the presence of which of the following specifiers?

A. Atypical features.
B. Melancholic features.
C. Catatonic features.
D. Diurnal variation.
E. None of the above.

**The correct response is option A: Atypical features.**

Interpersonal rejection insensitivity, increased appetite, and hypersomnia indicate the presence of atypical features (option A). Melancholic features (option B) are inability to respond to pleasurable stimuli, terminal insomnia, anorexia, excessive guilt, diurnal variation (worse in morning), and marked psychomotor symptoms. Catatonic features (option C) would include somnolence and waxy flexibility. Diurnal variation (option D), characterized by mood worse in the morning, is a feature of depression with melancholic features, but it is not in itself a specifier for mood episodes. **(pp. 158–159)**

6.11 What is the lifetime prevalence for major depression?

A. 3%.
B. 10%.
C. 17%.
D. 38%.
E. >50%.

**The correct response is option C: 17%.**

The National Comorbidity Study reported a lifetime prevalence of nearly 17% for major depression (option C). **(p. 160)**

6.12 Major depressive disorder has been associated with all the following pathophysiological abnormalities *except*

A. Increased rapid eye movement (REM) sleep latency.
B. Volumetric reductions of subgenual prefrontal cortex.
C. Decreased slow-wave sleep.

D. Blunting of growth hormone output in response to insulin challenge.

E. Abnormal suppression of cortisol following dexamethasone administration.

**The correct response is option A: Increased rapid eye movement (REM) sleep latency.**

Patients with major depressive disorder tend to have decreased REM sleep latency rather than increased REM sleep latency (option A). Options B–E describe pathophysiological abnormalities that have all been associated with major depressive disorder. **(pp. 161–163)**

6.13    Which of the following medications is *least* appropriate for the treatment of acute mania?

A. Carbamazepine.
B. Lithium.
C. Second-generation antipsychotic.
D. Gabapentin.
E. Valproate.

**The correct response is option D: Gabapentin.**

All the options except for gabapentin (option D) have been shown effective for the treatment of mania. Nearly all second-generation antipsychotics (option C) are approved to treat acute mania, and several have received indications for maintenance treatment of bipolar disorder or as adjuncts to lithium or valproate. **(pp. 164, 489–494)**

6.14    Which of the following is a first-line treatment for depression?

A. Second-generation antipsychotic.
B. Selective serotonin reuptake inhibitor (SSRI).
C. Tricyclic antidepressant.
D. Monoamine oxidase inhibitor (MAOI).
E. Intranasal ketamine.

**The correct response is option B: Selective serotonin reuptake inhibitor (SSRI).**

Treatment should typically start with one of the SSRIs because they are well tolerated and safe in overdose (option B). Low dosages are generally effective, and frequent dosage adjustments are usually unnecessary. The older tricyclic antidepressants (option C) and MAOIs (option D) are effective, but their use is limited by their side effects and concerns for safety in overdose, thus making them second-line treatment options. Intranasal ketamine (option E) is reserved for treatment-resistant depression. **(pp. 164–166, 472–489)**

6.15    Brexanolone can be used to treat which of the following?

A. Disruptive mood dysregulation disorder.
B. Postpartum depression.
C. Major depressive disorder.
D. Bipolar I disorder.
E. Schizoaffective disorder.

**The correct response is option B: Postpartum depression.**

Brexanolone is a GABA-receptor modulator that is U.S. Food and Drug Administration (FDA) approved for the treatment of postpartum depression and is administered by injection (option B). Patients must be enrolled in a federally mandated monitoring program to receive the medication. It is not approved for the treatment of the other disorders listed in options A and C–E. **(p. 166)**

6.16    A 30-year-old man with major depressive disorder has not responded to several trials of antidepressants. His insurer has approved the use of intranasal esketamine, which is FDA approved for treatment-refractory depression. Which of the following side effects could your patient experience from the use of the drug?

A. Dissociation.
B. Memory impairment.
C. Nausea and vomiting.
D. Scalp discomfort.
E. Hoarseness and cough.

**The correct response is option A: Dissociation.**

Although side effects can occur with any treatment, intranasal esketamine has the potential to induce dissociation (option A). Electroconvulsive therapy has been associated with memory impairment (option B). SSRI antidepressants often cause mild gastrointestinal side effects (option C). Scalp discomfort is reported to occur with repetitive transcranial magnetic stimulation (option D). Vagal nerve stimulation can cause hoarseness, cough, and dysphagia (option E). **(pp. 166–167, 477–478, 505–506)**

## — CHAPTER 7 —

# Anxiety Disorders

7.1    A 7-year-old girl is brought to a therapist by her parents because she refuses to attend school. She has pretended to be sick ("Mommy, my tummy hurts") several times a week for the past month to avoid going to school. She reports fear of being away from her mother during the day and has nightmares of "bad accidents" happening to her mother. Which of the following is the most likely diagnosis?

   A. Generalized anxiety disorder.
   B. Social anxiety disorder.
   C. Separation anxiety disorder.
   D. Panic disorder.
   E. Specific phobia.

   **The correct response is option C: Separation anxiety disorder.**

   Patients with separation anxiety disorder show developmentally inappropriate anxiety about being apart from an attachment figure, and children with this disorder may show school avoidance (option C). Patients with generalized anxiety disorder (option A) have pervasive anxiety about multiple life areas. Social anxiety disorder (option B) is a generalized or circumscribed anxiety about social situations. Patients with panic disorder (option D) have brief spells of intense anxiety and autonomic hyperarousal. Patients with a specific phobia (option E) have intense anxiety in response to a specific stimulus. In this case, school phobia is a symptom of separation anxiety rather than a specific phobia. **(pp. 169–172, 174, 179, 187)**

7.2     A teacher asks the parents of a 10-year-old boy to meet with her. She reports that since the boy started at the school 2 months ago, he has barely said a word and participates minimally in classroom activities. The parents report that, on the contrary, the boy is very talkative at home, and they haven't noticed any areas of concern. Which of the following is the most likely diagnosis?

A. Generalized anxiety disorder.
B. Social anxiety disorder.
C. Separation anxiety disorder.
D. Selective mutism.
E. Specific phobia.

**The correct response is option D: Selective mutism.**

The child portrayed in this vignette appears to have selective mutism (option D). This disorder is characterized by a persistent failure to speak in a situation in which speaking is expected when speech is normal in certain other environments, such as the home. People with separation anxiety disorder (option C) show age-inappropriate anxiety about being apart from an attachment figure, and children may show school avoidance. People with generalized anxiety disorder (option A) have pervasive anxiety about multiple life areas. Social anxiety disorder (option B) is a generalized or circumscribed anxiety about social situations; however, this patient's failure to speak is more characteristic of selective mutism. Patients with a specific phobia (option E) have intense anxiety in response to a specific stimulus. **(pp. 169–170, 172–174, 187)**

7.3     What is the primary fear that underlies social anxiety disorder?

A. Social situations.
B. Intimacy.
C. Sexual inadequacy.
D. Public humiliation.
E. Narcissistic injury.

**The correct response is option D: Public humiliation.**

Social anxiety is based on a fear of public embarrassment (option D), and for that reason, the fear of social situations (option A) is secondary to this. These persons also commonly fear performance situations such as public speaking, eating in restaurants, writing in front of other persons, or using public restrooms. Sometimes the fear becomes generalized, so that phobic persons avoid most social situations. Impaired intimacy (option B) and feelings of sexual inadequacy (option C) may occur in socially phobic persons, but they are not the primary motivating fear. Narcissistic injury (option E) is not associated with social anxiety disorder, but rather occurs when narcissists are deprived of something to which they feel entitled. **(pp. 174–176, 418)**

7.4 What is the typical age at onset for social anxiety disorder?

A. Preschool years.
B. Elementary school age.
C. Adolescence.
D. Early adulthood.
E. Middle adulthood.

**The correct response is option C: Adolescence.**

Social anxiety disorder begins during adolescence, and almost always before age 25 (option C). Specific phobias often have an onset in childhood. **(p. 176)**

7.5 All but which of the following medication classes is effective in treating social anxiety disorder?

A. Selective serotonin reuptake inhibitors (SSRIs).
B. Monoamine oxidase inhibitors (MAOIs).
C. Tricyclic antidepressants (TCAs).
D. β-Blockers.
E. Benzodiazepines.

**The correct response is option C: Tricyclic antidepressants (TCAs).**

Several SSRIs have a U.S. Food and Drug Administration (FDA) indication to treat social anxiety disorder (option A). The MAOIs and benzodiazepines (options B, E) are likely effective but are second-line choices because of their side effects and, in the case of benzodiazepines, their propensity for abuse. TCAs are probably less effective (option C), and socially anxious patients may be overly sensitive to their activating side effects (e.g., jitteriness). β-Blocking drugs (option D) are effective for the short-term treatment of performance-related anxiety but are otherwise ineffective for social anxiety disorder. **(p. 178)**

7.6     A 24-year-old woman presents to the emergency department complaining of the sudden onset of shortness of breath, dizziness, diaphoresis, chest pain, and a sense of impending doom. Her medical workup is negative, and her symptoms resolve within 30 minutes. She has had multiple previous episodes and fears her next spell. She avoids public places for fear of having an episode in public. Which of the following is the most likely diagnosis?

A. Generalized anxiety disorder.
B. Specific phobia.
C. Panic disorder.
D. Separation anxiety disorder.
E. Social anxiety disorder.

**The correct response is option C: Panic disorder.**

The patient in this vignette is presenting with classic symptoms of panic disorder (option C), as well as reporting multiple previous panic attacks and preoccupation with having subsequent attacks. Panic attacks typically peak within 10 minutes. Agoraphobia typically develops in response to panic attacks, so specific phobia (option B) is not the primary diagnosis. Patients with separation anxiety disorder (option D) show age-inappropriate anxiety about being apart from an attachment figure, and children with this disorder may show school avoidance. Patients with generalized anxiety disorder (option A) have pervasive anxiety about multiple life areas. Social anxiety disorder (option E) is a generalized or circumscribed anxiety about social situations. **(pp. 174, 179–187)**

7.7     Which of the following medications is the best long-term treatment option for specific phobia?

A. Fluoxetine.
B. Lorazepam.
C. Sertraline.
D. Alprazolam.
E. None of the above.

**The correct response is option E: None of the above.**

Benzodiazepines provide short-term relief from specific phobia. Long-term use is not recommended because of habituation and abuse potential. Otherwise, medications are not generally effective treatments for specific phobia. Patients can benefit from cognitive-behavioral therapy. A patient might be exposed to feared situations or objects through the techniques of systematic desensitization and flooding. Patients tend not to improve unless they are willing to confront feared situations or objects. **(pp. 178–179)**

7.8    Which two psychiatric disorders are the most likely to be comorbid with panic disorder?

A. Generalized anxiety disorder and major depressive disorder.
B. Generalized anxiety disorder and social anxiety disorder.
C. Major depressive disorder and alcohol use disorder.
D. Specific phobia and alcohol use disorder.
E. Persistent depressive disorder and generalized anxiety disorder.

**The correct response is option C: Major depressive disorder and alcohol use disorder.**

The most common comorbid psychiatric disorders are major depressive disorder and alcohol use disorder (option C). Major depressive disorder occurs in up to half of the patients with panic disorder and may be severe. Misuse of alcohol or other drugs complicates panic disorder in about 20% of the cases and may start in an attempt at self-medication. This complication is important to keep in mind when evaluating patients who abuse substances, because they may also have an underlying, treatable anxiety disorder. A person with panic disorder may also have another anxiety disorder requiring evaluation and treatment, such as social anxiety disorder or generalized anxiety disorder. **(p. 182)**

7.9    What substance has been implicated in the "false suffocation alarm" theory of panic disorder?

A. Carbon dioxide ($CO_2$).
B. Oxygen.
C. Sodium lactate.

D. Melatonin.

E. Carbon monoxide.

**The correct response is option A: Carbon dioxide ($CO_2$).**

Although the etiology of panic disorder is unknown, the observation that exposure to 5% $CO_2$ induces panic attacks has led to the "false suffocation alarm" theory (option A). The theory posits that patients with panic disorder are hypersensitive to $CO_2$ because they have an overly sensitive brain stem suffocation alarm system that produces respiratory distress, hyperventilation, and anxiety. **(p. 183)**

7.10   A 20-year-old college student develops symptoms of intense anxiety, racing heart, dizziness, diaphoresis, and shortness of breath. The symptoms resolve within less than 30 minutes. Prior to developing these symptoms, he had consumed several cups of coffee to help him stay up late to study for an examination. He has had no previous episodes. Which of the following is the most likely diagnosis?

A. Panic disorder.

B. Specific phobia.

C. Social phobia.

D. Substance-induced anxiety disorder.

E. Generalized anxiety disorder.

**The correct response is option D: Substance-induced anxiety disorder.**

This student portrayed in the vignette most likely has a caffeine-induced anxiety disorder because his panic symptoms appear attributable to the physiological effects of caffeine and not panic disorder (option D). The patient does not have symptoms of the other anxiety disorders listed in options A–C and E. **(p. 191)**

7.11   What is the literal meaning of the term *agoraphobia*?

A. Fear of people.

B. Fear of crowds.

C. Fear of open spaces.

D. Fear of the marketplace.

E. Fear of enclosed spaces.

**The correct response is option D: Fear of the marketplace.**

Agoraphobia's Greek roots mean "fear of the marketplace" (option D). In fact, a fear of the marketplace is not the primary problem for those with agoraphobia, although many individuals will describe a fear of shops and markets. Rather, the central problem is being separated from one's source of security. **(p. 187)**

7.12    A 30-year-old woman is meeting with her new family physician and reports feeling "wound up" all the time. She describes herself as a "worrier" and feels like she has always been this way. She tends to worry and ruminate about everything ("my health, my husband's health, our finances") but also reports insomnia and muscle tension in her neck and shoulders. She has a hard time concentrating. She drinks one cup of coffee in the morning but otherwise does not use stimulants. She denies being depressed or using alcohol or street drugs. Which of the following is the most likely diagnosis?

A. Separation anxiety disorder.
B. Generalized anxiety disorder.
C. Substance-induced anxiety disorder.
D. Agoraphobia.
E. Panic disorder.

**The correct response is option B: Generalized anxiety disorder.**

Patients with generalized anxiety disorder have a chronic tendency to worry and to feel on edge much of the time; they may have trouble concentrating, muscle tension, and insomnia (option B). Worries tend to center on realistic concerns, such as health or finances, but are difficult to control. Separation anxiety (option A) is the tendency to have intense anxiety about separation from an object of attachment. The patient in this scenario does not drink enough caffeine to account for substance-induced anxiety disorder (option C). Agoraphobia (option D) is fear of being in public places, and some patients find it very difficult to leave home. Panic disorder (option E) involves having recurrent panic attacks and a secondary fear of having subsequent attacks. **(pp. 169–170, 179, 186–191)**

7.13 Which of the following medications can be effective in treating generalized anxiety disorder in addition to individual psychotherapy?

A. Buspirone.
B. Escitalopram.
C. Venlafaxine.
D. Duloxetine.
E. All the above.

**The correct response is option E: All the above.**

Generalized anxiety disorder is usually treated with a combination of individual psychotherapy and medication. All medications listed as options are FDA approved to treat the disorder (option E). Patients should be educated about the chronic nature of the disorder and the tendency of symptoms to wax and wane, often in response to external stressors that the patient may be experiencing, such as family or marital problems. Cognitive-behavioral therapy may help the patient to recognize and control anxiety symptoms. Relaxation training, re-breathing exercises, and meditation can be easily taught and may be effective, especially if the condition is mild. Benzodiazepines should be avoided because of their tendency to induce tolerance and dependence. Their use in these patients should be limited. **(p. 190)**

—— CHAPTER 8 ——

# Obsessive-Compulsive and Related Disorders

8.1 Which of the following is *not* considered an obsession according to DSM-5?

A. Recurrent concerns about germs or contamination.
B. Fixation on the appearance of a particular body part.
C. Intrusive and disturbing thoughts about a loved one being murdered.
D. Obsessive desire to achieve ambitious career goals.
E. Need to collect worthless items and being unable to throw things away.

**The correct response is option D: Obsessive desire to achieve ambitious career goals.**

Obsessions are recurrent and persistent ideas, thoughts, impulses, or images that are experienced as intrusive and inappropriate and that cause marked anxiety or distress. This contrasts with the layman's usage of the term *obsession*. Option D is not an obsession because it is not experienced as intrusive and inappropriate. Options A, B, C, and E are consistent with major categories of obsessions: contamination, somatic, aggression, and hoarding, respectively. **(pp. 194–196)**

8.2 Which of the following behaviors is *not* considered a compulsive ritual?

A. Handwashing.
B. Counting.
C. Gambling.

D. Checking.

E. Symmetrical arranging.

**The correct response is option C: Gambling.**

Options A, B, D, and E are common compulsions. Compulsions are repetitive and intentional behaviors (or mental acts) performed in response to obsessions or according to certain rules that must be applied rigidly. Compulsions are meant to neutralize or reduce discomfort or to prevent a dreaded event or situation. The rituals are not connected in a realistic way to the event or situation or are clearly excessive. None of these descriptors apply to gambling, which is voluntary and perceived as pleasurable (option C). Gambling disorder, commonly referred to as "compulsive gambling," is classified as an addictive disorder rather than as an obsessive-compulsive disorder (OCD). **(pp. 194–197, 370–372)**

8.3   A 34-year-old man with generalized anxiety disorder tells his psychiatrist that he is worried that he may have OCD after reading an article on the Internet. He checks his door locks several times each morning before leaving for work, but this has never made him late for work. He worries that burglars could enter the house, but he is able to put the thought out of his mind after leaving his home. He has had these behaviors since adolescence. There is no family history of OCD. Based on this information, what should the psychiatrist tell this patient?

A. "We should start clomipramine immediately to target your OCD."

B. "OCD is not likely, based on the age at onset of your symptoms."

C. "OCD is not likely, based on your negative family history."

D. "OCD is not likely because your symptoms are so mild."

E. "OCD is not likely, based on your established diagnosis of generalized anxiety disorder."

**The correct response is option D: "OCD is not likely because your symptoms are so mild."**

This patient does not have OCD because his symptoms are mild and do not significantly interfere with his functioning (option D). Many psychiatrically healthy individuals have simple rituals such as checking locks. Compulsive behaviors should occupy a significant amount of time (1 hour a day or more) for a diagnosis of OCD. Age at onset and family history (options B, C) are not listed as part of the diagnostic criteria. Generalized anxiety disorder is often comorbid with OCD; thus, option E does not eliminate the possibility of an OCD diagnosis, but mild obsessive-compulsive symptoms do. Finally, clomipramine, although an effective medication for OCD, is not prescribed to people without the disorder (option A). **(pp. 194–197, 200)**

8.4  A 25-year-old man sees a psychiatrist for help with his OCD. He spends 2–3 hours each day arranging his bookshelves at home and is fed up with his need to do this. He feels that he is unable to stop his behavior and is afraid to have people over to his home for fear they might "mess up" the shelves. He has never sought treatment because he thought that he could handle it on his own. Which of the following is the best treatment strategy for this patient?

A. Clomipramine.
B. Fluoxetine.
C. Cognitive-behavioral therapy.
D. Fluoxetine plus cognitive-behavioral therapy.
E. Family therapy.

**The correct response is option D: Fluoxetine plus cognitive-behavioral therapy.**

The preferred treatment for OCD is the combination of an effective medication plus cognitive-behavioral therapy (option D). The selective serotonin reuptake inhibitor (SSRI) fluoxetine (option B) is effective, as are other SSRIs, and several are U.S. Food and Drug Administration (FDA) approved to treat OCD. Clomipramine (option A), a tricyclic antidepressant that is a relatively specific serotonin reuptake blocker, is also FDA approved to treat OCD. Because of its many side effects, it is used less frequently than the SSRIs. Typically, higher dosages of the SSRIs are needed to treat OCD than to treat major depression, and response is often delayed. Cognitive-behavioral therapy (option C) for OCD involves exposure and response prevention. For example, a patient might be exposed to a dreaded situation, event, or stimulus by various techniques (e.g., imaginal exposure, systematic desensitization, flooding) and then prevented from carrying out the compulsive ritual that usually results (e.g., handwashing after touching a doorknob). Family therapy (option E) may be helpful in educating family members about how best to interact with their relative with OCD but is adjunctive and does not replace medication or cognitive-behavioral therapy. **(p. 200)**

8.5    A patient presents to establish care with a new psychiatrist for treatment of OCD. He has seen several psychiatrists and therapists in the past 10 years, but he is frustrated because none of the treatments has been curative. How should the psychiatrist respond to this patient's concern?

   A. Review the patient's adherence to specific medications.
   B. Ask how long the patient has been able to stay in exposure therapy.
   C. Recommend a new medication.
   D. Inform the patient that OCD tends to be chronic.
   E. None of the above.

**The correct response is option D: Inform the patient that OCD tends to be chronic.**

OCD is chronic in nearly all cases; therefore, patients should not expect treatments to be curative (option D). Once it has been established that the goal of treatment is to reduce symptoms and improve quality of life rather than provide a cure, options A–C all become reasonable next steps. **(pp. 197–198)**

8.6    Which of the following disorders appears to be genetically linked with OCD?

   A. Pediatric autoimmune neuropsychiatric disorders associated with streptococcal infections (PANDAS).
   B. Tourette's disorder.
   C. Epilepsy.
   D. Huntington's disease.
   E. Sydenham's chorea.

**The correct response is option B: Tourette's disorder.**

OCD has a considerable genetic component as shown in family and twin studies, and it is linked with Tourette's disorder (option

B). PANDAS (option A) is an acquired form of OCD that occurs in children following group A β-streptococcal infection. Epilepsy, Huntington's disease, and Sydenham's chorea have been associated with OCD, but there is no evidence for a genetic link (options C–E). **(p. 198)**

8.7 A 17-year-old girl is brought to a psychiatrist by her concerned parents. She spends significant amounts of time staring at her nose in the mirror and has been saving her money for a rhinoplasty. The patient says that her nose is ugly and that her classmates stare at it, making fun of her through coded references. She cannot be reassured by her family that her nose looks normal and is even attractive. On examination, the nose appears unremarkable. She reports feeling demoralized by her concerns about her nose but has no history of depression, and she is not psychotic. There is no evidence of a thought disorder. Which of the following is the best diagnosis?

A. OCD with somatic obsessions.
B. Obsessive-compulsive personality disorder.
C. Delusional disorder, somatic type.
D. Body dysmorphic disorder.
E. Schizophrenia.

**The correct response is option D: Body dysmorphic disorder.**

Patients with body dysmorphic disorder are preoccupied with an imagined defect or flaw in physical appearance (option D). Because of this belief, body dysmorphic disorder should be the primary diagnosis in this case and not delusional disorder, somatic type (option C). The latter involves a delusional belief about bodily functions or sensations rather than physical appearance. Because of the circumscribed nature of her symptoms, body dysmorphic disorder is a better diagnosis than OCD with somatic obsessions (option A). Patients who have obsessive-compulsive personality disorder have a rigid, perfectionistic pattern of behavior (option B), but this usually has nothing to do with body concerns. Apart from her somatic preoccupation, this patient does not have symptoms to suggest schizophrenia such as auditory or visual hallucinations, bizarre behavior, or a thought disorder (option E). **(pp. 116–119, 124–125, 194–196, 199–202)**

8.8 A 30-year-old man sees a psychiatrist at his wife's insistence. She is concerned about the possibility of him having OCD after watching a TV show about hoarding. He has an extensive video game collection that he started at age 7. His collection is neatly arranged on shelves that do not take up much space. He is proud of his collection, and he would never think about getting rid of a single title because he sees no reason to do so. He enjoys playing video games for an hour or so each day, but otherwise keeps busy with work. He is tight with money and insists on doing many household chores himself because he believes that his family can never do the chores to his exacting standards. He has rigid political views that he happily shares with others on a social networking site. He does not feel that he has a significant problem with depression or anxiety. Which of the following is the most likely diagnosis?

A. OCD.
B. Obsessive-compulsive personality disorder.
C. Hoarding disorder.
D. Internet gaming disorder.
E. Marital discord (e.g., partner-relational problem).

**The correct response is option B: Obsessive-compulsive personality disorder.**

This patient's attitude toward his collecting behavior is not consistent with hoarding disorder, which requires that hoarding result in clutter that compromises the active use of living area (option C). His rigid, perfectionistic personality, however, is consistent with obsessive-compulsive personality disorder (option B), which is an important part of the differential diagnosis of OCD (option A) and related disorders. Because the patient is not bothered by his symptoms and finds enjoyment in his collecting, OCD is not a reasonable choice (option A). Internet gaming disorder, a variant of Internet addiction, is not a reasonable choice. It is not a DSM-5 diagnosis nor does the vignette imply that his Internet use is excessive (option D). The patient and his wife may have marital problems that center around his collection, but that does not explain his behavior (option E). **(pp. 199, 202–204, 337)**

8.9 What kind of psychotherapy is recommended for trichotillomania?

A. Supportive psychotherapy.
B. Habit reversal therapy.

C. Psychodynamic psychotherapy.
D. Interpersonal psychotherapy.
E. Acceptance and commitment therapy.

**The correct response is option B: Habit reversal therapy.**

Treatment of trichotillomania, or hair-pulling disorder, consists of medication combined with habit reversal therapy (option B). With habit reversal therapy, patients learn to identify when their hair pulling occurs (it is often automatic) and to substitute benign behaviors such as squeezing a ball. Some patients benefit from learning to apply barriers to prevent hair pulling, such as wearing gloves or a hat. Research shows that these techniques can be effective. All the other psychotherapies listed (options A, C–E) might be helpful but are not recommended for treating trichotillomania. **(p. 206)**

8.10    Which tricyclic antidepressant has shown benefit for trichotillomania?

A. Imipramine.
B. Doxepin.
C. Clomipramine.
D. Amitriptyline.
E. Nortriptyline.

**The correct response is option C: Clomipramine.**

Clomipramine has been shown to reduce hair-pulling behavior in those with trichotillomania (option C). It works preferentially through the serotonin system. The other medications (options A, B, D, E) are tricyclic antidepressants that are effective in treating major depressive disorder. **(p. 206)**

8.11    A 31-year-old woman has many open and bleeding sores on her forearms. She has sought help from dermatologists, who have prescribed various creams, all to no avail. The last dermatologist insisted that the woman seek a psychiatric evaluation. Which of the following is the most likely diagnosis?

A. Trichotillomania.
B. Unspecified obsessive-compulsive and related disorder.
C. Excoriation disorder.

D. Delusional disorder, somatic type.

E. OCD.

**The correct response is option C: Excoriation disorder.**

Excoriation (skin-picking) disorder is new to DSM-5 (option C). People with this disorder repetitively and compulsively pick at their skin, which leads to tissue damage. There are significant clinical similarities between excoriation disorder and trichotillomania (option A), and the criteria for the two disorders are similar. In rare cases, stimulants can cause skin-picking behaviors; therefore, stimulant use or abuse needs to be ruled out. Dermatological conditions such as scabies, atopic dermatitis, psoriasis, and blistering skin disorders also need ruling out. Patients with excoriation disorder are not delusional, and they do not pick in response to worrisome thoughts, thus ruling out both delusional disorder (option D) and OCD (option E). Option B is not reasonable because it is a diagnosis of exclusion. **(pp. 117–119, 194, 205–207)**

8.12 In excoriation disorder, what is the most common site for skin picking?

A. Face.

B. Hands.

C. Feet.

D. Arms.

E. Torso.

**The correct response is option A: Face.**

The face is the most common site of picking (option A). Other areas such as the hands, fingers, torso, arms, and legs are also common targets (options B–E). People with this disorder use their fingernails, knives, and even tweezers and pins for picking. Picking may result in significant tissue damage and may lead to medical complications such as localized infections or septicemia. **(p. 207)**

# ── CHAPTER 9 ──

# Trauma- and Stressor-Related Disorders

9.1    A 7-year-old boy is brought to a child psychiatrist by his new fos-
       ter parents. He had been removed from his biological parents'
       custody at an early age because of neglect, and he has been in
       several foster homes. His foster parents report that he is sullen
       and rarely smiles. He often becomes irritable, and they are un-
       able to console him. He appears to interact normally with his
       peers. Which of the following is the most likely diagnosis?

       A. Posttraumatic stress disorder (PTSD).
       B. Autism spectrum disorder.
       C. Reactive attachment disorder.
       D. Adjustment disorder with depressed mood.
       E. Disinhibited social engagement disorder.

       **The correct response is option C: Reactive attachment disorder.**

       Reactive attachment disorder can develop in children exposed to
       severe neglect (option C). These children do not seek caregiver
       attention as would their peers, nor do they respond to caregiver
       attempts to comfort them. Disinhibited social engagement disor-
       der (option E) involves inappropriate and overly familiar behav-
       ior with relative strangers, violating the social boundaries of the
       culture. The other options are not reasonable. PTSD (option A)
       involves hypervigilance, avoidance, and reexperiencing symp-
       toms that develop in response to a trauma, symptoms that the
       child does not have. Autism spectrum disorder (option B) is an
       important part of the differential of reactive attachment disorder,
       but its cardinal symptoms (deficits in social communication, re-

petitive patterns of behavior) are not present in this vignette. Adjustment disorder with depressed mood (option D) is diagnosed when someone develops mild depressive symptoms in reaction to a stressful event. Given this child's background and presenting symptoms, a diagnosis of reactive attachment better fits the picture than an adjustment disorder (option C). **(pp. 209–211, 213, 224)**

9.2    A 6-year-old girl is brought to a child psychiatrist by her new foster parents. She had been taken from her biological parents' custody at an early age because of neglect, and she has been in multiple previous foster homes. Since moving to her new home, her foster parents have noticed that she will initiate conversations with strangers at the supermarket. She once attempted to go home with another family. During the interview, the child jumps on the psychiatrist's lap and begins stroking her back. Testing has shown that she has a mild intellectual disability, and there is no history of a mood disorder. Which of the following is the best diagnosis?

A. PTSD.
B. Intellectual disability.
C. Bipolar I disorder.
D. Adjustment disorder with depressed mood.
E. Disinhibited social engagement disorder.

**The correct response is option E: Disinhibited social engagement disorder.**

Disinhibited social engagement disorder occurs when a neglected child behaves toward adults in an overly familiar fashion (option E). PTSD (option A) involves hypervigilance, avoidance, and reexperiencing symptoms that develop in response to a trauma, symptoms that the child does not have. Adjustment disorder with depressed mood (option D) occurs when someone develops mild depressive symptoms in reaction to a stressful event and for that reason is not a plausible response. There is no evidence of a bipolar disorder (option C), although bipolar patients may be disinhibited when manic or hypomanic. Although disinhibited social engagement disorder is often associated with cognitive delay, intellectual disability does not explain the child's behavior (option B). **(pp. 211–213, 224)**

9.3 Which of the following is the most common precipitating event for women diagnosed with PTSD?

A. Natural disaster.
B. Experiencing a fire.
C. Physical or sexual assault.
D. Hospitalization in an intensive care unit.
E. Combat.

**The correct response is option C: Physical or sexual assault.**

Physical or sexual assault is the most common precipitating event for women diagnosed with PTSD (option C). Most men with the disorder have experienced combat (option E). Response options A, B, and D can also lead to PTSD, but they are not the most common stressors for women with the disorder. **(p. 218)**

9.4 Which of the following symptom clusters is *not* required for a PTSD diagnosis?

A. Presence of intrusion symptoms associated with the traumatic event(s).
B. Dissociative reactions such as derealization or depersonalization.
C. Persistent avoidance of stimuli associated with the traumatic event(s).
D. Negative alterations in cognitions and mood.
E. Marked alterations in arousal and reactivity.

**The correct response is option B: Dissociative reactions such as derealization or depersonalization.**

Dissociative reactions can occur, as one manifestation of intrusion symptoms, but are not required for the PTSD diagnosis (option B). DSM-5 includes a specifier ("with dissociative symptoms") for patients with these symptoms. Symptoms in options A and C–E are required for the diagnosis of PTSD. **(pp. 213–215)**

9.5 Which of the following is the best medication choice for PTSD?

A. Sertraline.
B. Venlafaxine.

C. Diazepam.
D. Prazosin.
E. Lithium.

**The correct response is option A: Sertraline.**

Selective serotonin reuptake inhibitors (SSRIs), such as sertraline, are first-line treatments for PTSD (option A). Venlafaxine (option B) might be effective but is less well researched. Prazosin (option D) is often prescribed for PTSD-related nightmares but was no better than placebo in a large randomized controlled trial. Lithium (option E), effective for treating bipolar disorder, has no role in the treatment of PTSD. Benzodiazepines such as diazepam (option C) might be helpful for the short-term management of accompanying anxiety, but their long-term use should be avoided because of their potential for habituation and abuse. **(pp. 219–220, 489)**

9.6    Which of the following statements is true of eye movement desensitization and reprocessing (EMDR) therapy?

A. It is effective for treating adjustment disorders.
B. It is effective in reducing PTSD symptoms by providing patients skills to control anxiety and counter dysfunctional thoughts.
C. Research suggests that its efficacy is driven by exposure carefully integrated with eye movements.
D. Research suggests that its efficacy is driven by the exposure component.
E. Research suggests that its efficacy is driven by the eye movements.

**The correct response is option D: Research suggests that its efficacy is driven by the exposure component.**

Some experts recommend EMDR therapy for PTSD, but research suggests that its efficacy is driven by its exposure component, not eye movements (options C–E). Supportive psychotherapy is the treatment of choice for adjustment disorder (option A), and EMDR has no role in its treatment. Cognitive-behavioral therapy is effective in reducing PTSD symptoms by providing patients skills to control anxiety and counter dysfunctional thoughts (option B). **(pp. 220, 226)**

9.7 A 24-year-old man seeks the help of a psychiatrist because of problems with irritability and feeling "on guard" since a motor vehicle accident 2 weeks earlier. Luckily, he sustained only minor physical injuries, but his vehicle was destroyed. Since the accident, he has felt out of sorts and has developed intrusive memories and nightmares about the event. He has been using public transportation to get to work and now avoids going by the scene of the accident. Which of the following is the most likely diagnosis?

A. PTSD.
B. Acute stress disorder.
C. Adjustment disorder with anxious features.
D. Unspecified anxiety disorder.
E. None of the above.

**The correct response is option B: Acute stress disorder.**

The key difference between acute stress disorder and PTSD is duration of symptoms. PTSD (option A) is diagnosed when the symptoms have been ongoing for more than 1 month. Hypervigilance, avoidance, and reexperiencing that occur for the first month following a traumatic experience should be diagnosed as acute stress disorder (option B). The major difference between these diagnoses and adjustment disorder is that with adjustment disorder (option C), the patient develops depressive or anxious symptoms in reaction to a non-life-threatening event, such as a relationship breakup. Option D is not appropriate because it is a diagnosis of exclusion. **(pp. 220–223)**

9.8 A 17-year-old boy whose parents divorced 2 months earlier is brought to a therapist by his mother. He has always been a good student, but his grades have dropped, and he has been getting into fights at school over the past month. There is no history of behavioral problems. He says that he isn't depressed, and there have been no changes in his appetite, sleep, or activity level. He answers "I don't know" to most of the therapist's questions. Which of the following is the most likely diagnosis?

A. PTSD.
B. Acute stress disorder.
C. Adjustment disorder.
D. Major depressive disorder.
E. Reactive attachment disorder.

**The correct response is option C: Adjustment disorder.**

Acute behavioral changes following an identifiable stressor are suggestive of an adjustment disorder (option C). DSM-5 specifies five
subtypes, and this boy fits "with mixed disturbance of emotions and
conduct." Among adolescents, school problems are the most frequent stressors leading to an adjustment disorder, but parental separation and divorce are also common stressors. There has been no
threatened death, serious injury, or sexual violence, thus excluding
PTSD and acute stress disorder (options A, B). The patient reports
that he is not depressed, and no vegetative symptoms of depression
are described in the vignette, so major depressive disorder is not a
reasonable choice (option D). Reactive attachment disorder is a diagnosis for children who experience severe neglect who do not
show normal attention-seeking behavior directed toward their care-
givers, so option E is not plausible. **(pp. 210, 213, 223–227)**

9.9 Which of the following is the most likely stressor for adults with
adjustment disorder?

A. Separation or divorce.
B. Motor vehicle accident.
C. Sexual assault.
D. Terrorist attack.
E. Torture.

**The correct response is option A: Separation or divorce.**

Separation or divorce (option A) is a common stressor that can
lead to an adjustment disorder. The other stressors listed (options
B–E) are potentially life-threatening and could lead to the development of PTSD or acute stress disorder and thus are not plausible responses. **(p. 225)**

9.10 Which of the following is required for a diagnosis of adjustment
disorder?

A. A stressor.
B. Depressive symptoms.
C. Anxious symptoms.
D. Disturbance of conduct.
E. None of the above.

**The correct response is option A: A stressor.**

Without an identifiable stressor, there is no adjustment disorder (option A). The pertinent question for the clinician is, "What is the patient having trouble adjusting to?" Adjustment disorders are common, particularly in hospital settings. They can manifest in many ways such as with a disturbance of mood, anxiety, or a conduct disturbance (options B–D). **(pp. 223–224, 226)**

9.11 Which of the following is the best treatment for an adjustment disorder?

A. Sedative-hypnotics.
B. SSRIs.
C. Second-generation antipsychotics.
D. Supportive psychotherapy.
E. Cognitive-behavioral therapy.

**The correct response is option D: Supportive psychotherapy.**

Adjustment disorders typically resolve within 6 months of termination of the stressor; therefore, time and supportive psychotherapy are treatment mainstays (option D). A sedative-hypnotic (option A) might be helpful if the patient has insomnia as part of the adjustment disorder, but its use should last only days or weeks. Second-generation antipsychotics (option C) have no role in the treatment of adjustment disorders. If the patient has developed psychotic symptoms such as hallucinations or delusions, the patient does not have an adjustment disorder! SSRIs and cognitive-behavioral therapy (options B, E) might be useful but are probably not necessary because most adjustment disorders are short-lived and tend to remit. At some point, an adjustment disorder with depressed mood could evolve into a major depressive disorder, in which case antidepressant medication or cognitive-behavioral therapy might be indicated. **(pp. 226–227)**

# —CHAPTER 10—

# Somatic Symptom Disorders and Dissociative Disorders

10.1 A 30-year-old man presents to his primary care physician with a new concern that he could have a brain tumor. He reports that for the past week he has had tingling on his scalp. He had a mild headache the day before that resolved with ibuprofen. At his last visit a few months ago, he was concerned that he had pancreatic cancer because he noticed a small area of yellow discoloration on his upper arm. Which of the following is the most likely diagnosis?

A. Somatic symptom disorder.
B. Illness anxiety disorder.
C. Factitious disorder.
D. Conversion disorder.
E. Malingering.

**The correct response is option B: Illness anxiety disorder.**

Patients with illness anxiety disorder are preoccupied with the possibility of having or acquiring a serious illness based on mild or absent somatic symptoms (option B). In DSM-IV, many of these patients would have received a diagnosis of *hypochondriasis*. Patients with somatic symptom disorder (option A) are preoccupied with their somatic symptoms rather than the possibility that they might have a significant illness. Patients with factitious disorder (option C) feign illness in order to play the patient role. Patients who malinger (option E) feign illness for personal gain. (In DSM-5, malingering is categorized as a "V/Z code" condition that is not attributable to a mental disorder.) Conversion disorder (option D) is an alteration of voluntary motor or sensory function inconsistent with neurological disease, such as paralysis or abnormal movements. **(pp. 231, 233–237, 241, 243–244)**

10.2 A 24-year-old woman is referred for a neurology consultation for evaluation of spells that began 2 months earlier. She reports having "seizures" two or three times a week characterized by bilateral arm flapping without impairment of consciousness or loss of bowel or bladder control. The electroencephalogram is negative for epileptiform activity. Routine laboratory studies are unremarkable. Which of the following is the most likely diagnosis?

A. Somatic symptom disorder.
B. Convulsive disorder.
C. Factitious disorder.
D. Conversion disorder.
E. Malingering.

**The correct response is option D: Conversion disorder.**

The patient in this vignette best fits the diagnosis of conversion disorder, which involves altered voluntary motor or sensory function that is incompatible with known neurological or medical conditions (option D). Her spells are often referred to as *pseudoseizures*, although a more descriptive and less pejorative term is *nonepileptic seizures*. That is, they resemble seizures but are unaccompanied by abnormal brain waves and are considered a form of conversion disorder. Somatic symptom disorder (option A) is defined by the presence of excessive thoughts, feelings, or behaviors associated with somatic symptoms. The vignette does not suggest symptom falsification, as in factitious disorder (option C), or intentional production of symptoms, such as occurs in malingering (option E). Nor does the vignette suggest that the patient has a convulsive disorder (option B) because neither the electroencephalogram nor the clinical presentation suggests the presence of true seizures. **(pp. 230, 236–244)**

10.3 What is the minimum number of symptoms required for a diagnosis of somatic symptom disorder?

A. One.
B. Two.

C. Four.
D. Six.
E. Eight.

**The correct response is option A: One.**

The diagnosis of somatic symptom disorder requires the presence of one or more somatic symptoms that are distressing or result in significant disruption of daily life (option A). This represents a simplification of the more cumbersome DSM-IV construct of *somatization disorder,* in which eight symptoms spread across four categories were required. **(p. 230)**

10.4 A 60-year-old man receiving disability benefits sees his family physician in follow-up for chronic pain. He reports pain in multiple joints and often requests higher dosages of his opioid pain medication for better pain relief. Diagnostic studies show only changes consistent with normal aging. The patient's primary concern is with pain, and there is no evidence that he misuses his medications. He has been amenable to trying interventions such as physical therapy or cognitive-behavioral therapy, although they have not led to improvement in his pain. Which of the following is the most likely diagnosis?

A. Pain disorder.
B. Somatic symptom disorder.
C. Opioid use disorder.
D. Conversion disorder.
E. Malingering.

**The correct response is option B: Somatic symptom disorder.**

Patients who would have been diagnosed with pain disorder in DSM-IV now receive the more general diagnosis of somatic symptom disorder (option B). The specifier "with predominant pain" may be used to differentiate this condition from other manifestations of somatic symptom disorder. Although the patient requests pain medication, information in the vignette is insufficient to support a diagnosis of opioid use disorder (option C) or to suggest that he is feigning symptoms, as in malingering (option E). Conversion disorder (option D) involves symptoms that suggest a neurological condition, such as weakness or paralysis. **(pp. 230–231, 236, 243–244)**

10.5    A 19-year-old man presents to his family physician, convinced
        that his intestines are rotting and that he may already be dead.
        He is not able to cite any symptoms that give rise to this convic-
        tion. Physical examination and routine laboratory tests are nor-
        mal. The patient does not accept his physician's reassurance that
        he is healthy. Which of the following is the most likely diagnosis?

        A. Somatic symptom disorder.
        B. Illness anxiety disorder.
        C. Schizophrenia.
        D. Malingering.
        E. Unspecified somatic symptom disorder.

        **The correct response is option C: Schizophrenia.**

        In the differential diagnosis of somatic symptom disorder, psy-
        choses including schizophrenia need to be ruled out. In this vi-
        gnette, the patient is reporting bizarre delusions that could be
        due to schizophrenia (option C). A patient with illness anxiety
        disorder (option B) is preoccupied with having an illness but is
        not delusional. A patient with somatic symptom disorder (op-
        tions A, E) would be preoccupied with one or more symptoms
        rather than a conviction. Because there is no reason to believe
        that the patient is feigning illness, we can rule out malingering
        (option D). **(pp. 230, 233, 235–236, 243–244)**

10.6    A psychiatrist is asked to consult on a 25-year-old man admitted
        to a neurological service for sudden onset of lower-extremity
        weakness. The patient reports that he is unable to walk, although
        diagnostic studies have not shown any physical reason for the
        symptoms. The patient asks if he will ever get any better. How
        should the psychiatrist respond?

        A. "Your condition will most likely improve with time."
        B. "You will most likely be permanently disabled."
        C. "Your prognosis is guarded."
        D. "It is too early to draw any conclusion."
        E. "It will depend on your willingness to engage in cognitive-
           behavioral therapy."

        **The correct response is option A: "Your condition will most
        likely improve with time."**

Conversion symptoms are common in hospitals, and follow-up studies show that most individuals with conversion symptoms tend to improve or remit spontaneously (option A). Onset may occur at any point throughout life. A favorable outcome is generally associated with acute onset, a precipitating stressor, good premorbid adjustment, and the absence of medical or neurological comorbidity. There are no established treatments for conversion disorder. (pp. 237–239)

10.7   A 55-year-old woman sees her family physician for an annual physical examination. During a symptom review, she reports chronic dyspepsia. She had the same complaint during her last three visits. A medical workup for her symptom was negative 3 years ago. She is not preoccupied with this symptom, and her social and occupational functioning is normal. The physician considers diagnosing somatic symptom disorder because there is no obvious medical explanation for her complaint. Her medical student, fresh from a psychiatry clerkship, objects and says that it would be inappropriate. Why so?

A. Patients with somatic symptom disorder must have multiple somatic complaints.
B. The patient's lack of interest in her symptoms makes a conversion disorder more likely.
C. The physician has not investigated possible motivations for secondary gain or to play the patient role.
D. The diagnosis of somatic symptom disorder requires the patient to have significant preoccupation or personal investment in his or her symptoms.
E. The medical student is wrong, and it is appropriate to diagnose this patient with somatic symptom disorder.

The correct response is option D: The diagnosis of somatic symptom disorder requires the patient to have significant preoccupation or personal investment in his or her symptoms.

Somatic symptom disorder requires the presence of excessive thoughts, feelings, or behaviors related to the symptom or symptoms, and the woman in the vignette has none of these (option D). Only one symptom is required for somatic symptom disorder (option A), but the patient has no abnormal health concerns, and conversion disorder requires a functional neurological symptom (option B), which she does not have. For these reasons, neither response option is appropriate. Also, there is no evidence that the woman is feigning her symptoms or is motivated to play the patient role (option C). The astute medical student should be congratulated for speaking up! **(pp. 230–231, 236)**

10.8    Which of the following is the recommended treatment for somatic symptom disorder?

A. Selective serotonin reuptake inhibitors.
B. Benzodiazepine tranquilizers.
C. Regularly scheduled visits with the same physician.
D. Referral to specialists in order to provide higher levels of care.
E. Aggressive medical workups to offer greater reassurance to patients.

**The correct response is option C: Regularly scheduled visits with the same physician.**

Patients with somatic symptom disorder should have regularly scheduled visits with the same physician to provide reassurance and continuity of care (option C). This will reduce the likelihood that the patient will undergo unnecessary and irrelevant diagnostic studies and procedures (options D, E). Antidepressants (option A) have no established role in the treatment of somatic symptom disorders, apart from illness anxiety disorder. Long-term use of benzodiazepines (option B) is not recommended because of the potential for habituation and abuse. **(pp. 238–239)**

10.9    A psychiatrist is asked to see a 25-year-old man with chronic renal failure admitted to a general medical floor for complications resulting from poor compliance with recommended dialysis. He shows a fair understanding of his medical condition but says that he just feels like taking a day off from dialysis every now and then. Further evaluation shows no evidence of an underlying depression, anxiety disorder, cognitive impairment, psychosis, or personality disorder. Which of the following is the most likely diagnosis?

A. Psychological factors affecting other medical conditions.
B. Factitious disorder.
C. Malingering.

D. Unspecified depressive disorder.

E. Somatic symptom disorder.

**The correct response is option A: Psychological factors affecting other medical conditions.**

The essential feature of psychological factors affecting other medical conditions is the presence of one or more clinically significant psychological or behavioral factors that adversely affect the medical condition by increasing the risk for suffering, death, or disability (option A). These factors can include psychological distress, patterns of interpersonal interaction, coping styles, and maladaptive health behaviors (such as denying symptoms or poor adherence to medical recommendations). Unlike a somatic symptom disorder (option E), these patients must have a clear medical diagnosis. In this vignette, there is no evidence of motivation to play the patient role or for personal gain, making factitious disorder and malingering (options B, C) unlikely. Option D is inappropriate because no evidence of depression was found. **(pp. 239–241, 243–244)**

10.10 A psychiatrist is asked to see a 25-year-old man with chronic renal failure admitted to a general medical floor for complications resulting from poor compliance with recommended dialysis. He has demanded to leave against medical advice. He has been threatening and verbally abusing staff members. He has fair understanding of his medical condition and is not delirious or confused. Which of the following is the best explanation for his behavior?

A. Psychological factors affecting other medical conditions.

B. Malingering.

C. Unspecified depressive disorder.

D. Somatic symptom disorder.

E. Personal choice in the absence of a mental disorder.

**The correct response is option E: Personal choice in the absence of a mental disorder.**

Not all poor decisions are due to mental illness! Regardless of the seriousness of their medical condition, some patients will simply make bad decisions (option E). No evidence has been presented to implicate psychological factors affecting the man's medical condition (option A). In addition to lacking a motivation to play the patient role, or being preoccupied with his symptoms, his disorder is medically valid, thus ruling out malingering and somatic symptom disorder (options B, D). Option C is a poor choice because the vignette does not provide evidence of a depressive disorder. **(pp. 231, 239–240, 243–244)**

10.11 A 10-year-old boy receives several new video games for his birthday. The following day he tells his mother that he does not feel up to going to school because of stomach upset, although he appears well. His mother gives him a thermometer to check his temperature and leaves the room. When she comes back, the thermometer shows a temperature of 112°F. Which of the following is the most likely diagnosis?

A. Factitious disorder.
B. Malingering.
C. Somatic symptom disorder.
D. Separation anxiety disorder.
E. Psychological factors affecting other medical conditions.

**The correct response is option B: Malingering.**

The boy in this example is most likely feigning illness to stay home from school to play video games. Rubbing a thermometer (usually against a blanket or similar object) is one method used to fake a fever, although in this case the boy does not realize that 112°F is a preposterous temperature elevation! Feigning illness for personal gain constitutes malingering (option B). Feigning illness to occupy the sick role is consistent with factitious disorder (option A). No evidence suggests that the boy is avoiding school because of fear of parental separation, which would suggest a separation anxiety disorder (option D). Patients with somatic symptom disorder (option C) are preoccupied with one or more somatic symptoms present 6 or more months, symptoms that do not fit the vignette. The diagnosis of psychological factors affecting other medical conditions (option E) requires the presence of a specific medical condition and is not a plausible response. **(pp. 169–170, 230, 239–241, 243–244)**

10.12 Which personality disorder is frequently comorbid with dissociative identity disorder?

A. Schizotypal personality disorder.
B. Schizoid personality disorder.
C. Dependent personality disorder.
D. Borderline personality disorder.
E. Narcissistic personality disorder.

**The correct response is option D: Borderline personality disorder.**

Patients with dissociative identity disorder often meet criteria for
other mental disorders. Borderline personality disorder, found in
up to 70% of patients with dissociative identity disorder, is diagnosed based on the person's history of mood instability, identity
disturbance, deliberate self-harm, and other symptoms characteristic of the disorder (option D). The other personality disorders listed (options A–C, E) can occur but are much less frequent
in these patients. **(p. 247)**

10.13 What is the standard treatment for depersonalization/derealiza-
tion disorder?

A. A benzodiazepine.
B. Fluoxetine.
C. A second-generation antipsychotic.
D. Cognitive-behavioral therapy.
E. There is no standard treatment.

**The correct response is option E: There is no standard treatment.**

There is no standard treatment for depersonalization/derealiza-
tion disorder (option E). A controlled trial showed that fluoxetine
(option B) was ineffective. A benzodiazepine (option A) might
lessen the anxiety that accompanies the disorder, but it is not a
treatment for the disorder itself. Patients have been reported to
benefit from cognitive-behavioral therapy (option D) and hypno-
sis, but these options are not standard treatments. There is no established role for antipsychotics in treating this condition (option
C). **(pp. 252–253)**

10.14 A 19-year-old college student reports that for the past 2 weeks, since smoking cannabis for the first time, she has felt cut off from herself. She feels that she is watching herself go through the motions and feels unable to connect with her experiences. She did not feel this way before smoking cannabis. Which of the following is the best diagnosis?

A. Dissociative identity disorder.
B. Depersonalization/derealization disorder.
C. Dissociative amnesia.
D. Substance-induced mood disorder.
E. Schizophrenia.

**The correct response is option B: Depersonalization/derealization disorder.**

Patients with depersonalization/derealization disorder often feel disconnected from their experiences and/or surroundings (option B). This experience can occur in the course of another mental disorder (e.g., major depressive disorder), but the information provided in this vignette does not suggest one. Depersonalization/derealization disorder is sometimes preceded by the use of a substance such as marijuana, but substance-induced mood disorder (option D) is not an appropriate diagnosis because the complaints are of dissociation, not a mood disorder. Patients with dissociative identity disorder (option A) report feeling disconnected from reality, but this is because of their perception of having many personality states, or alters. Dissociative amnesia (option C) refers to the inability to recall important autobiographical information that is not attributable to ordinary forgetfulness. The patient is not reporting hallucinations or delusions, so schizophrenia is not a plausible option (option E). **(pp. 122, 245, 249, 251–253)**

10.15 A 35-year-old man presents to the emergency department. He shows the staff his driver's license and requests help because he has forgotten who he is and where he lives. His driver's license shows that he lives in a town more than 100 miles away. A medical workup including brain imaging is unremarkable. Neuropsychological assessment shows gaps in his ability to recall autobiographical information, but formal testing of memory is normal. Which of the following is the most likely diagnosis?

A. Dissociative identity disorder.
B. Depersonalization/derealization disorder.
C. Dissociative amnesia.
D. Posttraumatic stress disorder.
E. Factitious disorder.

**The correct response is option C: Dissociative amnesia.**

The man is exhibiting a classic dissociative fugue, a diagnosis now classified in DSM-5 as a subtype ("with dissociative fugue") of dissociative amnesia (option C). The critical feature is that the person is unable to recall his or her past and assumes a new identity, which may be partial or complete. Fugues usually involve sudden, unexpected travel away from home or one's workplace, are not due to a dissociative identity disorder (option A), and are not induced by a substance or a general medical condition such as temporal lobe epilepsy. Fugue states are reported to occur in psychologically stressful situations, such as natural disasters, war, or personal rejections. Dissociative symptoms can occur in posttraumatic stress disorder but not in fugue states; furthermore, in posttraumatic stress disorder, the stressful event involves exposure to actual or threatened death (option D). The patient in this vignette is not feigning illness in order to play the patient role (option E), nor does he appear disconnected from his current experiences and/or surroundings (option B). **(pp. 213, 241, 249–251)**

# —CHAPTER 11—

# Feeding and Eating Disorders

11.1 A mother reports to a pediatrician that her 4-year-old son has been eating small quantities of dirt and pebbles from the garden at home. Which of the following is the most likely diagnosis?

A. Pica.
B. Rumination disorder.
C. Avoidant/restrictive food intake disorder.
D. Other specified feeding disorder.
E. None of the above.

**The correct response is option A: Pica.**

Pica is a pattern of eating nonnutritive substances on a persistent basis for at least 1 month (option A). Rumination disorder (option B) involves regurgitating swallowed food in the absence of a gastrointestinal disorder that would cause the disturbance. Patients with avoidant/restrictive food intake disorder (option C) have limited food intake rather than a propensity to eat nonnutritive substances. The symptoms described in the vignette clearly meet criteria for pica, so it would be incorrect to use an "other specified" or "unspecified" feeding disorder diagnosis (option D). **(pp. 255–257)**

11.2 A mother reports to a pediatrician that her 15-month-old daughter mouths on a variety of inanimate objects in the home. Which of the following is the most likely diagnosis?

A. Pica.
B. Rumination disorder.

C. Avoidant/restrictive food intake disorder.

D. Other specified feeding disorder.

E. None of the above.

**The correct response is option E: None of the above.**

The daughter appears to be exhibiting normal developmental behavior in that she is mouthing objects and is younger than 2 years (option E). She does not fit the criteria for an unspecified or other specified feeding or eating disorder (option D), nor is she swallowing regurgitated food (option B). Pica (option A) is not an appropriate diagnosis because the child is older than 2 years, and there is no evidence that the child is consuming a nonnutritive substance. Patients with avoidant/restrictive food intake disorder (option C) have limited food intake rather than a propensity to eat nonnutritive substances. **(pp. 255–257)**

11.3  A 7-year-old girl is brought to a pediatric gastroenterologist by her parents. They are concerned because they have noticed that she has been regurgitating swallowed food and then swallowing it again or sometimes expelling it. The girl does not report symptoms such as heartburn or stomach pain. Her food intake is appropriate for her age, and she does not appear preoccupied with her body shape or size. A medical workup is unremarkable. Which of the following is the most likely diagnosis?

A. Pica.

B. Rumination disorder.

C. Avoidant/restrictive food intake disorder.

D. Bulimia nervosa.

E. Anorexia nervosa.

**The correct response is option B: Rumination disorder.**

The girl has rumination disorder, which is characterized by the repeated regurgitation of food (option B). The disorder occurs across age ranges and in both genders. Individuals with this disorder repeatedly regurgitate swallowed or partially digested food, which may then be re-chewed and either re-swallowed or expelled. Adolescents and adults are less likely to re-chew regurgitated material than are younger children. This child does not have body image concerns that would characterize an eating disorder such as bulimia nervosa (option D) and anorexia nervosa (option E) or a pattern of restrictive or avoidant eating behavior (option C), and she is not ingesting nonnutritive substances (option A). **(pp. 256, 257, 259)**

11.4 An 11-year-old boy with autism spectrum disorder is brought to a pediatrician because his mother is concerned about his poor appetite. He has always been a picky eater, but his mother is especially concerned because it's about time for his "growth spurt." The boy is thin but not emaciated and is of normal height. He tells his doctor that he's not very interested in food and that he finds the textures of most foods unappetizing. He denies being preoccupied with being thin, and there is no evidence of depression. Which of the following is the most likely diagnosis?

A. Pica.
B. Rumination disorder.
C. Avoidant/restrictive food intake disorder.
D. Bulimia nervosa.
E. Anorexia nervosa.

**The correct response is option C: Avoidant/restrictive food intake disorder.**

The boy in this vignette has an autism spectrum disorder and might have unusual eating habits consistent with the restricted range of interests seen in such patients. That said, the key difference between avoidant/restrictive food intake disorder (option C) and an eating disorder such as anorexia nervosa or bulimia nervosa (options D, E) is that patients with avoidant/restrictive food intake disorder do not have preoccupation with their body image. Pica (option A) is a pattern of eating nonnutritive objects as food. Rumination disorder (option B) involves regurgitating swallowed food in the absence of a gastrointestinal disorder that would cause the disturbance. **(pp. 255, 257–259)**

11.5 A 50-year-old man is brought to his family physician at his wife's insistence. She is concerned that he has lost 15 pounds in the past month and stopped going to work. He "barely eats a thing," she says. The man reports that he no longer has any interest in anything. He spends most of the day watching TV but does not pay much attention to the shows. He complains of poor sleep, waking up at about 3:00 A.M. every morning and not being able to go

back to sleep. He displays a restricted affect. Which of the following is the most likely diagnosis?

A. Pica.
B. Rumination disorder.
C. Avoidant/restrictive food intake disorder.
D. Major depressive disorder.
E. Anorexia nervosa.

**The correct response is option D: Major depressive disorder.**

The importance of this vignette is to highlight the fact that eating
disturbances are common throughout psychiatry, and major depressive disorder is one of the main causes of poor appetite and
weight loss. Thus, the patient's symptoms are consistent with a
classic major depressive episode (option D) rather than a primary disorder of feeding or eating. This patient is not ingesting
nonnutritive substances (option A), regurgitating swallowed
food in the absence of a disorder that would cause the disturbance (option B), or engaging in disturbed eating patterns because of a preoccupation with his body weight and shape (option
E). Avoidant/restrictive food intake disorder (option C) is not
appropriate because the symptoms are better explained by major
depressive disorder. **(pp. 149–154, 255–261)**

11.6   What is the key difference between anorexia nervosa and bulimia
       nervosa?

A. Presence of bingeing behavior.
B. Presence of purging behavior.
C. Preoccupation with one's body weight.
D. Current body weight.
E. Personality traits.

**The correct response is option D: Current body weight.**

Both disorders overlap and intertwine, but the fundamental difference is that patients with anorexia nervosa mainly restrict
their food intake, whereas bulimic patients have episodes of
binge-eating and purging. Although patients with anorexia are
significantly underweight, patients with bulimia tend to be of
near-normal weight (option D), even when their illness is active.

Both types of patients have an intense preoccupation with their body weight and shape (option C). Nonetheless, many anorexia patients have the binge-eating/purging subtype (options A, B) and engage in significant binge eating followed by compensatory behaviors. Importantly, patients with anorexia and bulimia tend to have different personality characteristics (option E), but this is not part of the DSM-5 criteria. Bulimic patients more commonly have "acting out" personality disorders, such as borderline personality disorder, than do anorexic patients. **(pp. 259–262)**

11.7    Which of the following physical examination findings is *not* typical of anorexia nervosa?

A. Tachycardia.
B. Hypokalemia.
C. Amenorrhea.
D. Hair loss.
E. Constipation.

**The correct response is option A: Tachycardia.**

Patients with poorly controlled anorexia nervosa develop bradycardia rather than tachycardia (option A). Options B–E are common abnormalities. **(Table 11–2 [Medical complications of the eating disorders], p. 266)**

11.8    Which brain region plays an important role in regulating feeding behavior?

A. Thalamus.
B. Hypothalamus.
C. Pineal gland.
D. Amygdala.
E. Entorhinal cortex.

**The correct response is option B: Hypothalamus.**

The hypothalamus has a central role in regulating feeding behavior (option B). With the neurotransmitter serotonin, the hypothalamus helps modulate feeding behavior by producing feelings of fullness and satiety. It is unclear if the other regions listed in options A and C–E play a role in eating disorders. **(p. 267)**

11.9    Which of the following physical examination findings would sug-
        gest a diagnosis of bulimia nervosa or the binge-eating/purging
        subtype of anorexia nervosa rather than another eating disorder?

A. Constipation.
B. Decreased thyroid-stimulating hormone.
C. Dental caries.
D. Amenorrhea.
E. Hair loss.

**The correct response is option C: Dental caries.**

Patients with eating disorders who induce vomiting are at risk
for serious dental problems, including erosion of tooth enamel
and multiple caries (option C). Esophageal erosion or tears
caused by the force of repeated vomiting can occur. Options A, B,
D, and E are not specific for purging behavior. **(p. 265)**

11.10   During a routine health maintenance examination, a 30-year-old
        man tells his family physician that he has been having trouble
        losing weight. He reports that three to four times each week, he
        loses control of his eating and consumes a large quantity of food
        such that he feels physically uncomfortable afterward. He is
        overweight and has some concern about his body image, but he
        denies being obsessed with being thin. He denies excessive exer-
        cise or other compensatory behaviors. Which of the following is
        the most likely diagnosis?

A. Binge-eating disorder.
B. Rumination disorder.
C. Avoidant/restrictive food intake disorder.
D. Bulimia nervosa.
E. Anorexia nervosa.

**The correct response is option A: Binge-eating disorder.**

The patient has binge-eating disorder, a diagnosis new to DSM-5
(option A). It is a diagnosis used for patients with recurrent spells
of binge eating who do not have the compensatory behavior that
is present in bulimia nervosa, such as purging (option D). Patients with avoidant/restrictive food intake disorder (option C)
avoid eating and do not have binges. Patients with rumination

disorder (option B) regurgitate swallowed food, but this is not a compensatory mechanism because these patients may re-swallow the regurgitated food, and they do not have episodic bingeing behavior. Many patients with binge-eating disorder are men, and most have a history of compensatory behaviors. An-orexia nervosa (option E) is not an appropriate response because the man has no significant weight loss. **(pp. 257, 259, 261–263)**

11.11 Which antidepressant is contraindicated in patients with eating disorders?

A. Fluoxetine.
B. Sertraline.
C. Bupropion.
D. Venlafaxine.
E. Mirtazapine.

**The correct response is option C: Bupropion.**

Bupropion (option C) is contraindicated in patients with active eat-ing disorders because it can lower the seizure threshold in patients with electrolyte disturbances. The other medications listed (op-tions A, B, D, E) can be safely used in these patients. **(pp. 269–270)**

11.12 Which medication is U.S. Food and Drug Administration (FDA) approved for the treatment of bulimia nervosa?

A. Sertraline.
B. Fluoxetine.
C. Lithium.
D. Venlafaxine.
E. Olanzapine.

**The correct response is option B: Fluoxetine.**

Fluoxetine is FDA approved for treatment of bulimia nervosa (option B). Other selective serotonin reuptake inhibitors (SSRIs), such as sertraline (option A), and serotonin-norepinephrine re-uptake inhibitors, such as venlafaxine (option D), may be benefi-cial as well, but they are not approved for bulimia treatment. Lithium (option C) and olanzapine (option E) have no role in the treatment of bulimia nervosa. **(pp. 269–270)**

11.13   What is the first objective in treating an eating disorder?

A. Correct faulty cognitions about body image.
B. Modify distorted eating behaviors.
C. Restore nutritional status.
D. Correct unhealthy home environment that gives rise to the disorder.
E. Initiate SSRI to address disturbed serotonergic neurotransmission.

**The correct response is option C: Restore nutritional status.**

In treating any eating disorder, the first order of business is to restore proper nutritional status (option C). This will help to correct electrolyte imbalances and restore a healthy body weight. The next objective is to modify distorted eating behaviors (option B). The third objective is to correct cognitive distortions about body image (option A). SSRIs may help with bulimia nervosa, but they have no clear role in the treatment of anorexia (option E). Family therapy can be a helpful part of treatment to address an unhealthy home environment, but this would come after addressing the other objectives (option D). **(pp. 268–271)**

# — CHAPTER 12 —

# Sleep-Wake Disorders

12.1 Which sleep stage is characterized by rapid conjugate eye movements, reduced muscle tone, and respiratory and cardiac rate fluctuations with loss of body temperature control?

A. Stage N1 (non–rapid eye movement [NREM] 1).
B. Stage N2 (NREM 2).
C. Stage N3 (NREM 3).
D. Stage R (REM).
E. All the above.

**The correct response is option D: Stage R (REM).**

REM sleep is characterized by rapid conjugate eye movements, reduced muscle tone, and respiratory and cardiac rate fluctuations with loss of body temperature control (option D). Stage N1 sleep (option A) marks the transition from wakefulness to sleep, and it is characterized by beta and slow theta waves. Stage N2 sleep (option B) is characterized by the appearance of sleep spindles and K complexes. Stage N3 sleep (or deep sleep) (option C) is characterized by delta waves. **(Table 12–2 [Sleep stages in adults], p. 275)**

12.2 Which procedure can be used to measure excessive daytime sleepiness?

A. Polysomnography.
B. Multiple Sleep Latency Test.
C. Electroencephalogram (EEG).
D. A sleep log.
E. Neuropsychological evaluation.

**The correct response is option B: Multiple Sleep Latency Test.**

The Multiple Sleep Latency Test is used to measure excessive daytime sleepiness (option B). Polysomnography (option A) can be used to assess narcolepsy, breathing-related sleep disorders, and REM sleep behavior disorder. EEG (option C) is a part of polysomnography. A sleep log (option D) may be used to record daytime naps but does not measure excessive sleepiness. A neuropsychological evaluation (option E) does not have a clearly defined role in the routine assessment of sleep disorders. **(p. 275)**

12.3   As part of a cognitive-behavioral approach to treating insomnia, which of the following is *not* a standard recommendation?

A. Discontinuing the intake of alcohol, caffeine, and sedative-hypnotics.
B. Avoiding reading, working, or watching TV in bed.
C. Staying awake in bed for long periods of time until sleep onset occurs.
D. Going to bed and waking up at the same time every day, even on weekends.
E. Avoiding napping.

**The correct response is option C: Staying awake in bed for long periods of time until sleep onset occurs.**

Patients should set limits on the amount of time spent in bed (option C). Options A, B, D, and E are standard recommendations. **(pp. 277–278)**

12.4   What is the treatment of choice for insomnia disorder?

A. Temazepam.
B. Trazodone.
C. Diphenhydramine.
D. Zolpidem.
E. Cognitive-behavioral therapy for insomnia (CBTi).

**The correct response is option E: Cognitive-behavioral therapy for insomnia (CBTi).**

CBTi is increasingly recognized as the treatment of choice for insomnia disorder (option E). Important elements include sleep restriction (limiting the amount of time in bed) and stimulus control (using the bed only for sleep). Any of the medications in options A–D can be used to treat transient and short-term insomnia, in combination with appropriate sleep hygiene. **(pp. 277–279)**

12.5    A 35-year-old man complains to his family physician of difficulty falling asleep for the past 8 months. It takes him up to an hour to fall asleep, and he reports feeling fatigued throughout the day. He sometimes feels irritable but denies significant depression. He does not snore, nor does he feel sleepy during the day. He stopped his caffeine intake a couple of months ago after reading about sleep hygiene on the Internet. Which of the following is the most likely diagnosis?

A. Hypersomnolence disorder.
B. Narcolepsy.
C. Insomnia disorder.
D. Obstructive sleep apnea.
E. Other specified insomnia disorder.

**The correct response is option C: Insomnia disorder.**

The man in this vignette has an insomnia disorder, defined as trouble initiating or maintaining sleep on a regular basis for at least 3 months (option C). Comorbid psychiatric or medical problems do not preclude this diagnosis. Patients with hypersomnolence disorder (option A) do not feel rested despite excessive sleep. Patients with obstructive sleep apnea (option D) have frequent arousals secondary to hypoventilation, resulting in daytime sleepiness. Patients with narcolepsy (option B) have the recurrent irrepressible need to nap, decreased REM sleep latency, hypocretin deficiency, and episodes of cataplexy. Other specified insomnia disorder (option E) is not appropriate because it is a diagnosis of exclusion. **(pp. 276–281, 283–284)**

12.6    Which of the following suggests hypersomnolence disorder rather than narcolepsy?

A. Daytime napping.
B. Decreased REM sleep latency.
C. Spells of brief loss of muscle tone (hypotonia).
D. Hypocretin deficiency.
E. Sleep drunkenness.

**The correct response is option E: Sleep drunkenness.**

Sleep drunkenness, or excessive grogginess after waking, is more characteristic of hypersomnolence disorder than narcolepsy (option E). Daytime napping (option A) occurs in both disorders. Hypocretin deficiency (option D) and spells of hypotonia (option C) are characteristic of narcolepsy rather than hypersomnolence disorder. Decreased REM sleep latency (option B) can be present in both disorders. **(pp. 280–282)**

12.7    A 22-year-old woman presents to a sleep disorders clinic. She reports that she is groggy most every morning, and it takes her more than an hour to become alert. She sleeps 9–10 hours at night. She feels sleepy during the day and will sometimes take a 1- to 2-hour nap. She denies episodes of cataplexy or excessive caffeine use. Which treatment may be effective for this patient?

A. Selective serotonin reuptake inhibitor (SSRI).
B. Benzodiazepine.
C. Stimulant.
D. Nonbenzodiazepine hypnotic.
E. Antihistamine.

**The correct response is option C: Stimulant.**

The woman in this vignette appears to have a hypersomnolence disorder, and stimulants such as methylphenidate are probably the most effective treatment (option C). They have the potential for abuse, and for that reason, their use needs careful monitoring. Improved sleep hygiene is also important. Scheduled napping may help as well. Antidepressants (option A) are not appropriate because no information suggests that the patient is depressed. A benzodiazepine, a nonbenzodiazepine hypnotic, or an antihistamine (options B, D, E) would only cause greater sedation and are therefore inappropriate. **(p. 280)**

12.8    What causes narcolepsy?

A. Loss of cholinergic cells in the nucleus basalis.
B. Loss of hypocretin-secreting cells in the hypothalamus.
C. Decrease in REM sleep latency.
D. Poor sleep hygiene.
E. The cause is unknown.

**The correct response is option B: Loss of hypocretin-secreting cells in the hypothalamus.**

Narcolepsy is one of the few DSM-5 disorders in which a biological mechanism has been identified (option E) and has been included in the criteria set. Narcolepsy nearly always results from the loss of hypothalamic hypocretin-producing cells (option B), causing cerebrospinal fluid hypocretin-1 deficiency (one-third or less of control values, or 110 pg/mL in most laboratories). (Hypocretin is a neurotransmitter that regulates arousal, wakefulness, and appetite.) As for the other response options, a decrease in REM sleep latency (option C) is a symptom of narcolepsy rather than its cause. Poor sleep hygiene (option D) does not lead to narcolepsy. Loss of cholinergic cells in the nucleus basalis (option A) is a finding associated with Alzheimer's disease. **(pp. 68, 281–283)**

12.9  Which of the following is an effective treatment for sleep attacks associated with narcolepsy?

A. Tricyclic antidepressant.
B. Sodium oxybate.
C. Methylphenidate.
D. Zolpidem.
E. Improved sleep hygiene.

**The correct response is option C: Methylphenidate.**

The clinical management of narcolepsy involves different treatments for the sleep attacks and the auxiliary symptoms. Stimulants such as methylphenidate (option C) or dextroamphetamine are the preferred drugs for treating sleep attacks because of their rapid onset and relative lack of side effects. Modafinil is an effective alternative to the stimulants. Sodium oxybate (option B) is approved by the U.S. Food and Drug Administration (FDA) for the treatment of cataplexy associated with narcolepsy and has been shown to reduce the frequency of cataplexy episodes. Tricyclic antidepressants (option A) are sometimes used to treat cataplexy or sleep paralysis but have little effect on sleep attacks. Zolpidem (option D) is an effective hypnotic but has no role in treating sleep attacks. Sleep hygiene (option C) should always be recommended to patients but will not treat sleep attacks. **(p. 283)**

12.10 What is the technical term used for a decrease in airflow during sleeping?

A. Apnea.
B. Hypopnea.
C. Cheyne-Stokes breathing.
D. Hyperventilation.
E. None of the above.

**The correct response is option B: Hypopnea.**

Hypopnea (option B) is a decrease in airflow. Apnea (option A) is a pause in breathing. Cheyne-Stokes breathing is a pattern of crescendo-descrescendo variation in tidal volume seen in central sleep apnea (option C). Hyperventilation is rapid breathing that is often related to anxiety (option D). **(pp. 283–284, 560)**

12.11 A 45-year-old obese man complains to his family physician of chronic trouble with sleep maintenance. He falls asleep easily at night but awakens 10–20 times throughout the night. He feels fatigued during the day and occasionally takes short naps. He says that his wife tells him that he snores loudly at times but not on most nights. He sleeps in a quiet dark room and goes to bed at about the same time on most nights but might stay up 30–45 minutes later than usual on weekends. His blood pressure is normal. He drinks two to three cups of coffee in the morning and may have a 12 oz can of soda in the late afternoon. What is the best next step in management of this patient?

A. Prescribe a benzodiazepine.
B. Have the patient eliminate caffeine intake.
C. Order a Multiple Sleep Latency Test.
D. Order a polysomnogram.
E. Counsel the patient on sleep hygiene and follow up in 3 months.

**The correct response is option D: Order a polysomnogram.**

The cause of this patient's sleeping problems is not entirely clear, but obstructive sleep apnea hypopnea needs to be ruled out with polysomnography (option D). Counseling the patient on appropriate sleep hygiene (option E) should also be done, but it is best to proceed with the polysomnography. Lifestyle changes alone are unlikely to have much of an effect, including eliminating caffeine intake (option B). If the patient has obstructive sleep apnea hypopnea, a continuous positive airway pressure (CPAP) machine would be the method of choice to help him with sleep rather than a benzodiazepine (option A) or a hypnotic. The Multiple Sleep Latency Test (option C) measures daytime fatigue, but in this case, polysomnography would provide more useful diagnostic information. **(pp. 275, 283–285)**

12.12 Which of the following is *not* suggestive of obstructive sleep apnea hypopnea?

A. Snoring.
B. Daytime fatigue.
C. Apneic episodes.
D. Crescendo-decrescendo variation in tidal volume.
E. Difficult-to-control hypertension.

**The correct response is option D: Crescendo-decrescendo variation in tidal volume.**

Crescendo-decrescendo variation in tidal volume is called *Cheyne-Stokes breathing*. This sort of breathing is characteristic of individuals who have central sleep apnea comorbid with heart failure, renal failure, or history of stroke (option D). Options A–C and E are characteristics associated with obstructive sleep apnea hypopnea. **(pp. 284–286)**

12.13 Which of the following treatment methods can be used for refractory cases of obstructive sleep apnea hypopnea?

A. Weight-loss counseling.
B. CPAP.
C. Sedative-hypnotics.
D. Respiratory assist devices.
E. Hypoglossal nerve stimulator.

**The correct response is option E: Hypoglossal nerve stimulator.**

A hypoglossal nerve stimulator is an implantable device that activates the genioglossus muscle, improving airway patency (option E). Respiratory assist devices (option D) are positive pressure airway devices that can provide a missed breath. They are used to treat central sleep apnea. Sedative-hypnotics (option C) should be avoided in obstructive sleep apnea hypopnea. CPAP (option B) and weight-loss counseling (option A) are first-line treatments for obstructive sleep apnea hypopnea. **(pp. 284–285)**

12.14 A 50-year-old woman who has chronic obstructive pulmonary disease reports to her family physician that she has morning headache and daytime fatigue. Routine laboratory studies are re-markable for elevated carbon dioxide ($CO_2$). A polysomnogram shows periods of decreased respiration. Which of the following is the most likely diagnosis?

A. Obstructive sleep apnea hypopnea.
B. Central sleep apnea.
C. Sleep-related hypoventilation.
D. Hypersomnolence disorder.
E. Narcolepsy.

**The correct response is option C: Sleep-related hypoventilation.**

Sleep-related hypoventilation is the result of a decreased re-sponse to high $CO_2$ during sleep and is characterized by frequent episodes of shallow breathing lasting longer than 10 seconds during sleep (option C). Polysomnography shows episodes of decreased respiration associated with elevated $CO_2$ levels. Sleep-related hypoventilation is usually associated with lung disease. Obstructive and central sleep apnea (options A, B) are character-ized by episodes of apnea and hypopnea on a polysomnogram. Central sleep apnea is caused by variable respiratory effort, and obstructive sleep apnea hypopnea is caused by upper airway re-sistance. Patients with hypersomnolence disorder (option D) sleep excessively and still do not feel rested. Narcolepsy (option E) is characterized by sleep attacks and episodes of cataplexy. **(pp. 278, 281, 283–288)**

12.15 A 27-year-old man who works nights at a convenience store re-ports to his family physician that his energy is chronically low and he has little motivation. He can only sleep 4–6 hours during the day. He tries to maintain a diurnal schedule on his days off on the weekend but has trouble falling asleep at night. Which of the following is the most likely diagnosis?

A. Insomnia disorder.
B. Obstructive sleep apnea hypopnea.
C. Hypersomnolence disorder.
D. Circadian rhythm sleep-wake disorder.
E. Narcolepsy.

**The correct response is option D: Circadian rhythm sleep-wake disorder.**

The man has the shift work type of circadian rhythm sleep-wake disorder (option D). Shift workers tend to have high rates of on-the-job sleepiness, tend to make cognitive errors, and have high rates of drug use and divorce. They may never feel fully rested. When they want to sleep, they cannot, and when they are expected to be awake and alert, they are sleepy and drowsy. As for the other response options, insomnia disorder (option A) is trouble initiating or maintaining sleep on a regular basis for at least 3 months. Patients with hypersomnolence disorder (option C) do not feel rested despite excessive sleep. Patients with obstructive sleep apnea hypopnea (option B) have frequent arousals secondary to hypoventilation, resulting in daytime sleepiness. Patients with narcolepsy (option E) have a recurrent, irrepressible need to nap, decreased REM sleep latency, hypocretin deficiency, and episodes of cataplexy. **(pp. 276, 278, 281, 284, 288–290)**

12.16 What is the best treatment for circadian rhythm sleep-wake disorder, shift work type?

A. Improved sleep hygiene.
B. Methylphenidate to improve alertness.
C. Zolpidem to assist with daytime sleep.
D. Melatonin to regulate circadian rhythm.
E. Discontinue shift work.

**The correct response is option E: Discontinue shift work.**

Unfortunately, for the man in the vignette above, the best option is to discontinue shift work (option E) and to resume a normal diurnal schedule. For most people, earning a paycheck often trumps such considerations. Even though improved sleep hygiene could help, it cannot override the deleterious effect of shift change. Interestingly, the stimulant drug armodafinil has been FDA approved to treat shift work disorder. Options A–D will not help correct the man's sleep disorder. **(p. 290)**

12.17 What is the DSM-5 diagnosis used for both sleepwalking and sleep terrors?

A. NREM sleep arousal disorder.
B. REM sleep behavior disorder.
C. Parasomnia.
D. Circadian rhythm sleep-wake disorder.
E. None of the above.

**The correct response is option A: NREM sleep arousal disorder.**

Sleepwalking and sleep terrors are both referred to as NREM sleep arousal disorders because they occur during Stage 3 of sleep (option A). REM sleep behavior disorder (option B) occurs during REM sleep. Parasomnia (option C) is a general term used for abnormal behavior or experiences that occur during sleep or sleep-wake transitions. Circadian rhythm sleep-wake disorders (option D) are persistent or recurring patterns of sleep disruption that result from an altered sleep-wake schedule or occur when the sleep-wake cycle is not correctly synchronized with a person's daily schedule. **(pp. 288, 290–292, 294)**

12.18 A 15-year-old boy has recurrent vivid dreams with frightening violent content. He wakes up in the morning with a racing heart and heavy breathing, but he does not scream or act out. Which of the following is the most likely diagnosis?

A. REM sleep behavior disorder.
B. NREM sleep arousal disorder, sleep terror type.
C. Nightmare disorder.
D. Parasomnia.
E. None of the above.

**The correct response is option C: Nightmare disorder.**

Nightmares are vivid, and patients may have some autonomic arousal on awakening, but they do not scream on awakening as do people with sleep terrors (option C). On a physiological level, nightmares occur during REM sleep, whereas sleep terrors occur during NREM sleep (option B). Parasomnia (option D) is a general term for abnormal experiences or behavior that occurs during sleep or sleep-wake transition. REM sleep behavior disorder (option A) is defined by the presence of arousal during REM sleep associated with vocalization and/or complex motor behaviors. **(pp. 290, 292–294)**

12.19 Which sleep disorder is associated with Parkinson's disease, Lewy body dementia, and multiple system atrophy?

A. REM sleep behavior disorder.
B. NREM sleep arousal disorder, sleep terror type.
C. Nightmare disorder.
D. Parasomnia.
E. Central sleep apnea.

**The correct response is option A: REM sleep behavior disorder.**

There is a relationship between REM sleep behavior disorder and neurodegenerative disorders (particularly Parkinson's disease, dementia with Lewy bodies, and multiple system atrophy; option A). At least 50% of individuals with REM sleep behavior disorder presenting in sleep clinics will eventually develop one of these conditions. The other responses (options B–E) are problematic disorders but are not associated with neurodegenerative disorders. **(pp. 294–295)**

12.20 A 31-year-old woman reports to her family physician that she has the uncomfortable sensation of having to move her legs at night when she is in bed. She says that she does not sleep well because of this. She wonders if something can be given to treat her condition. Which of the following can be used to treat this condition?

A. Zolpidem.
B. Pramipexole.
C. Sodium oxybate.
D. Clonazepam.
E. Imipramine.

**The correct response is option B: Pramipexole.**

The woman has restless legs syndrome, classified as a sleep-wake disorder in DSM-5 because it interferes with sleep and may be associated with periodic limb movements during sleep. The syndrome affects about 5% of the general population. Symptoms typically begin in the evening and are relieved by moving the legs or walking. The sensations can delay sleep or waken the person from sleep. Dopamine agonists such as pramipexole or ropinirole may be used to treat restless legs syndrome (option B). Options A and C–E are not treatments for restless legs syndrome. **(pp. 295–296)**

# —CHAPTER 13—

# Sexual Dysfunction, Gender Dysphoria, and Paraphilic Disorders

13.1 How long should a disorder of sexual function be present prior to diagnosis?

A. At least 18 months.
B. At least 4 months.
C. At least 1 month.
D. At least 6 months.
E. At least 1 year.

**The correct response is option D: At least 6 months.**

DSM-5 requires that disorders of sexual function be present for at least 6 months prior to diagnosis (option D). **(p. 301)**

13.2 Which of the following would preclude a diagnosis of a sexual dysfunction?

A. Severe relationship stress.
B. A nonsexual mental disorder that would account for symptoms.
C. Disturbance caused by substance use or medication.
D. Disturbance caused by medical condition such as diabetes.
E. Any of the above.

**The correct response is option E: Any of the above.**

Any of the items listed would preclude a diagnosis of a sexual dysfunction (option E). In addition to having persisted 6 months or longer, the disorder causes clinically significant distress. DSM-5 requires that the disorder is not due to severe relationship stress; another nonsexual mental disorder; or the effects of a substance, medication, or medical condition (options A–D) (e.g., diabetes mellitus). **(p. 301)**

13.3   A 22-year-old man reports to his family physician that he has had persistent difficulty achieving orgasm during intercourse with his partner. He has no trouble attaining an erection. The problem has been ongoing since the relationship began about a year ago. He does not have any difficulty achieving orgasm during masturbation and reports that otherwise his relationship is going well. He does not take any medications. Which of the following is the most likely diagnosis?

A. No diagnosis.
B. Other specified sexual dysfunction.
C. Delayed ejaculation.
D. Male hypoactive sexual desire disorder.
E. Erectile disorder.

**The correct response is option C: Delayed ejaculation.**

The fact that the problem occurs only during intercourse with a partner does not preclude a diagnosis of delayed ejaculation (option C). The patient denies problems achieving an erection, ruling out erectile disorder (option E), and nothing in the vignette indicates a problem with sexual desire (option D). The patient's difficulty as described does meet criteria for a more specific sexual dysfunction (option B). **(pp. 301–303, 308–309)**

13.4   A 28-year-old man reports to his family physician that he has had persistent difficulty achieving orgasm both with his partner and while masturbating. He has no trouble attaining an erection. His problem has been ongoing since the relationship began about a year ago. He reports that otherwise his relationship is going well. He takes fluoxetine but no other medication. Which of the following is the most likely diagnosis?

A. Medication-induced sexual dysfunction.
B. Other specified sexual dysfunction.
C. Delayed ejaculation.

D. Male hypoactive sexual desire disorder.

E. Erectile disorder.

**The correct response is option A: Medication-induced sexual dysfunction.**

Fluoxetine, along with the other selective serotonin reuptake inhibitors (SSRIs), can induce sexual dysfunction (option A). Typically, this consists of ejaculatory delay or failure in men. Even though the man reports delayed ejaculation (option C), he does not meet its criteria because it appears to be medication-induced. There is no information to suggest either low sexual desire or trouble obtaining erections (options D, E). Other specified sexual dysfunction (option B) is inappropriate because it is a diagnosis of exclusion. **(pp. 310–311)**

13.5 A 30-year-old woman reports to her family physician of ongoing sexual difficulties with her partner for the last several years. She experiences vaginal and pelvic pain during intercourse. She denies that there is difficulty achieving vaginal penetration, and she is not sure about tightening of her pelvic muscles during penetration. Which of the following is the most likely diagnosis?

A. Dyspareunia.

B. Vaginismus.

C. Genito-pelvic pain disorder.

D. Female sexual interest/arousal disorder.

E. None of the above.

**The correct response is option C: Genito-pelvic pain disorder.**

Genito-pelvic pain disorder is diagnosed when a person has pain or discomfort, muscular tightening, or fear about pain when having sexual intercourse (option C). This disorder reflects a change from DSM-IV, wherein two disorders—dyspareunia and vaginismus (options A, B)—were used to diagnose sexual pain disorders. They are now merged into a single category because clinicians had difficulty in distinguishing between the two, and their reliability was low. Female sexual interest/arousal disorder (option D) reflects a decreased interest in sexual activity rather than pain and difficulty with vaginal penetration. **(pp. 306–308)**

13.6 A 50-year-old man reports to his family physician that in the past few months he has had a new onset of erectile dysfunction during intercourse and masturbation. He is baffled about why it is happening at his age and reports that his sexual interest remains strong. He has been feeling more jittery than usual over the past few months, and he reports occasional palpitations and diaphoresis on review of systems. What is the next best step in management of this patient?

A. Refer to a psychiatrist.
B. Start an SSRI.
C. Refer to a psychotherapist.
D. Order thyroid-stimulating hormone test.
E. None of the above.

**The correct response is option D: Order thyroid-stimulating hormone test.**

Hyperthyroidism can cause late-onset erectile dysfunction, and the patient's other symptoms suggest hyperthyroidism (option D). Options A–C would not be helpful in uncovering the underlying etiology of the patient's complaint. **(p. 312; Table 13–3 [Causes of erectile disorder], p. 313)**

13.7 What medication can be used to treat premature ejaculation?

A. Sildenafil.
B. Alprostadil.
C. Vardenafil.
D. Paroxetine.
E. Tadalafil.

**The correct response is option D: Paroxetine.**

Medication now has a large role in treating the sexual dysfunctions. Paroxetine (option D) and other SSRIs have been used off-label to treat premature (early) ejaculation because a common side effect is ejaculatory delay. Men can also benefit from 1% dibucaine (Nupercaine) ointment applied to the coronal ridge and frenulum of the penis to reduce stimulation. Options A–C and E are used to treat erectile disorder. **(pp. 313–314)**

13.8    Which of the following medications is a standard treatment for
        erectile disorder?

   A. Vardenafil.
   B. Paroxetine.
   C. Dibucaine.
   D. Testosterone.
   E. Topical estrogen.

**The correct response is option A: Vardenafil.**

Vardenafil is one of the phosphodiesterase-5 inhibitors, which
are the first-line treatment for erectile disorder (option A). Paroxetine and dibucaine (options B, C) can be used to treat premature
ejaculation. Testosterone (option D) is sometimes given for low
sexual desire, but unless it is being used to treat hypogonadism,
the results are mixed. Topical estrogen has no role in treating
erectile disorder (option E). **(p. 314)**

13.9    Which of the following is *not* typical of gender dysphoria?

   A. Onset occurs in childhood.
   B. The child prefers to play with children of the same gender.
   C. The child expresses a strong desire to be rid of one's primary
      and secondary sexual characteristics because of incongruence
      between one's expressed and experienced gender.
   D. The child expresses strong preference for cross-sex roles in
      make-believe play.
   E. The child shows a strong preference for games, toys, and ac-
      tivities stereotypically associated with the opposite gender.

**The correct response is option B: The child prefers to play with
children of the same gender.**

In childhood, patients with gender dysphoria generally prefer to
play with children of the opposite gender (option B). Options A
and C–E are typical of gender dysphoria. **(pp. 315–317)**

13.10   A 40-year-old man reports to his psychiatrist that he enjoys
        dressing in women's clothing prior to intercourse, but this has
        caused conflict with his wife. He identifies himself as hetero-

---

sexual, and he reports that he is comfortable being male. Which of the following is the most likely diagnosis?

A. Gender dysphoria.
B. Transvestic disorder.
C. Voyeuristic disorder.
D. Exhibitionistic disorder.
E. Frotteuristic disorder.

**The correct response is option B: Transvestic disorder.**

Transvestic disorder is a paraphilia in which one becomes sexually aroused by dressing in the clothing of the opposite gender (option B). Patients with gender dysphoria (option A), by contrast, experience distress because of a perceived incongruence between their assigned and experienced genders. Patients with voyeuristic disorder (option C) become aroused by watching unsuspecting individuals when disrobing, naked, or engaged in sexual activity. Exhibitionistic disorder (option D) involves becoming aroused by exposing one's genitals to unsuspecting individuals, and frotteuristic disorder (option E) involves becoming sexually aroused from rubbing against a nonconsenting individual. **(pp. 315, 320–322; Table 13–5 [DSM-5 paraphilic disorders], p. 317; Table 13–6 [Paraphilic disorders], p. 319)**

13.11  What is the DSM-5 term for an anomalous sexual activity preference?

A. Paraphilic disorder.
B. Paraphilia.
C. Infantilism.
D. Infantilism disorder.
E. None of the above.

**The correct response is option B: Paraphilia.**

*Paraphilia* is the term used to describe anomalous sexual activity preference (option B). Paraphilic disorder (option A) refers to the distress experienced because of an anomalous sexual activity preference. Infantilism (option C) is a paraphilia in which the person obtains sexual arousal and gratification by behaving like an infant. Infantilism disorder (option D) is not a DSM-5 disorder. Infantilism should be coded as other specified paraphilic disorder. **(pp. 317–318; Table 13–6 [Paraphilic disorders], p. 319)**

13.12 Which of the following has *not* been used in the treatment of paraphilic disorders?

A. Masturbatory satiation.
B. SSRIs.
C. Behavioral activation.
D. Cognitive-behavioral therapy.
E. Couples therapy.

**The correct response is option C: Behavioral activation.**

Options A, B, D, and E are all methods that have been used in the treatment of paraphilic disorders. Cognitive-behavioral therapy (option D) has been used to restructure the faulty cognitions that people with paraphilic disorders use to justify their behaviors. Masturbatory satiation (option A) is used to satiate (or bore) the patient with his or her own deviant fantasies, whereas couples therapy (option E) is helpful for those in committed relationships. Behavioral activation (option C) is not used in patients with paraphilic disorders but rather is used in depressed patients to reverse their withdrawal and isolation. Although no medications have been approved for paraphilic disorders, SSRIs (option B) have been used to reduce paraphilic fantasies and behavior. **(pp. 322–323, 453)**

# —CHAPTER 14—

# Disruptive, Impulse-Control, and Conduct Disorders

14.1 A 7-year-old girl is brought to a therapist by her mother. Her mother says the girl is always touchy and irritable and gets very angry when told to do anything. The behavior has been present for more than a year. When asked about her symptoms, the girl says that it's her mother's fault for always making her mad. She has not engaged in any stealing, fire setting, or runaway behavior. She gets along with her peers, and her grades in school are good. Which of the following is the most likely diagnosis?

A. Antisocial personality disorder.
B. Conduct disorder.
C. Attention-deficit/hyperactivity disorder (ADHD).
D. Oppositional defiant disorder.
E. Normal development.

**The correct response is option D: Oppositional defiant disorder.**

Oppositional defiant disorder is characterized by irritable, angry, and defiant behavior that does not involve frank antisocial behavior (option D). Antisocial personality disorder (option A) is a diagnosis reserved for adults; children with antisocial behavior receive a diagnosis of conduct disorder (option B). Nothing in the vignette suggests ADHD, which is characterized by overactivity, inattention, and impulsivity (option C). Whereas most children are occasionally naughty, children with oppositional defiant disorder are more frequently naughty, and more so than most children at the same mental age (option E). **(pp. 326–328)**

14.2   A 16-year-old boy with an autism spectrum disorder is brought to the emergency department by his family. His father reports that he broke two windows and smashed several plates in the kitchen after his father told him that he would not be able to use the computer for the next day because he had failed to clean up his room. The boy has had similar destructive outbursts when his computer privileges have been restricted in the past. Ordinarily, he is quiet, keeps to himself, and does not bother others. He does not have a history of truancy, fire setting, cruelty to animals, or fighting. Which of the following is the most likely diagnosis?

A. Oppositional defiant disorder.
B. Conduct disorder.
C. Antisocial personality disorder.
D. Intermittent explosive disorder.
E. No additional diagnosis apart from autism spectrum disorder.

**The correct response is option D: Intermittent explosive disorder.**

Intermittent explosive disorder can be diagnosed in addition to an autism spectrum disorder if the outbursts are significant enough to merit clinical attention (option D). It appears that the outburst is not typical behavior for this child and occurs only in a circumscribed context, making oppositional defiant disorder and conduct disorder (options A, B) less credible diagnostic options. Antisocial personality disorder (option C) is a diagnosis reserved for adults. **(pp. 328–330)**

14.3   A 16-year-old boy is brought to a psychiatrist at his parents' insistence for problem behavior ongoing for 3 years. He has had repeated legal trouble for acts of vandalism, and he has been expelled from school several times for fighting. He is failing all his classes. He tells the psychiatrist that he doesn't care about his schoolwork and has no remorse for his actions. What DSM-5 specifier is appropriate for this form of conduct disorder?

A. With limited prosocial emotions.
B. With antisocial personality features.
C. With psychopathic personality features.

D.  Childhood-onset type.

E.  DSM-5 does not have a descriptor for such cases.

**The correct response is option A: With limited prosocial emotions.**

"With limited prosocial emotions" is the DSM-5 specifier used for children with conduct disorder who show no remorse or interest in meeting societal expectations (option A). This is the childhood equivalent of psychopathy. He would qualify for the specifier adolescent-onset type but not childhood-onset type (option D), which is for children whose conduct disorder has an onset prior to age 10 years. Options B and C have terms not used in DSM-5. **(pp. 331–333)**

14.4  A 35-year-old man is charged with arson after burning down a building he owned in order to collect insurance money. He has no previous criminal history, and his work history has been stable. He denies any previous episodes of fire setting. Which of the following options best explains his behavior?

A.  Antisocial personality disorder.

B.  There is no psychiatric diagnosis.

C.  Pyromania.

D.  Intermittent explosive disorder.

E.  Conduct disorder.

**The correct response is option B: There is no psychiatric diagnosis.**

Although setting a fire for material gain is a criminal act, it is not attributable to a psychiatric disorder (option B). In DSM-5, the man's act would be classified as the V/Z code condition "adult antisocial behavior," which is not discussed in the chapter. V/Z code conditions may be a focus of clinical attention but are not considered mental disorders. Persons with antisocial personality disorder (option A) and conduct disorder (option E) have an enduring pattern of antisocial behavior, and a single action is inconsistent with these constructs. Patients with pyromania (option C) have a recurrent compulsion to set fires, and they are not typically motivated by material gain. Intermittent explosive disorder (option D) is associated with recurrent behavioral outbursts, but that would not explain the man's behavior. **(pp. 328, 330, 334–335)**

14.5    What is the treatment for pyromania?

   A. Cognitive-behavioral therapy.
   B. Selective serotonin reuptake inhibitor (SSRI).
   C. Mood stabilizer such as carbamazepine.
   D. Second-generation antipsychotic such as risperidone.
   E. There is no standard treatment for pyromania.

**The correct response is option E: There is no standard treatment for pyromania.**

There is no standard treatment for pyromania (option E). Clinicians should begin by identifying co-occurring psychiatric disorders that could be a focus of treatment, such as major depressive disorder. Treatment of the co-occurring disorder may itself reduce fire-setting behavior. There is no clear role for medication in the treatment of pyromania. If the patient is a child or an adolescent, then the parents should be taught consistent but nonpunitive methods of discipline. Family therapy may help in dealing with the broader issue of family dysfunction often found in patients with pyromania. The patient needs to understand the dangerousness and significance of the fire setting. **(p. 335)**

14.6    A 24-year-old woman comes forward to establish care with a therapist. She reports a problem with compulsive stealing. She has taken small items of modest value from stores and from the homes of friends and family on many occasions since adolescence. She reports feeling tension before the theft and a sense of gratification afterward. She is motivated to change her behavior because she was recently given probation for shoplifting. She denies any other criminal activity or interpersonal problems. Which of the following is the most likely diagnosis?

   A. Conduct disorder.
   B. Antisocial personality disorder.
   C. Kleptomania.
   D. Compulsive shopping.
   E. Oppositional defiant disorder.

**The correct response is option C: Kleptomania.**

Kleptomania is compulsive stealing of objects of modest value (option C), and the stealing behavior does not occur in the context of a wider pattern of antisocial behavior as in conduct disorder (option A), a diagnosis applicable to children and adolescents, and antisocial personality disorder (option B). Compulsive shopping (option D) is not a reasonable option because the vignette notes that the woman steals items but does not buy them. Oppositional defiant disorder (option E) is a diagnosis for children who are irritable, defiant, and quick to anger but who do not regularly engage in behavior that infringes on the rights of others. (pp. 326, 330, 335–337)

14.7 All but which of the following might be beneficial for patients with intermittent explosive disorder?

A. Fluoxetine.
B. Oxcarbazepine.
C. Cognitive-behavioral therapy.
D. Benzodiazepine tranquilizers.
E. Fluoxetine and oxcarbazepine.

**The correct response is option D: Benzodiazepine tranquilizers.**

Benzodiazepines should be avoided because of their tendency to cause behavioral disinhibition (option D). Both fluoxetine (option A) and the antiepileptic drug oxcarbazepine (option B), and their combination (option E), have been found superior to placebo in reducing impulsive aggression in people with intermittent explosive disorder. Other SSRIs, mood stabilizers, and β-blockers have been used to treat the condition, but their use is supported mainly by case studies or small case series. Second-generation antipsychotics have been used to dampen aggressive impulses in other clinical populations and may be helpful in treating intermittent explosive disorder, but they have not been specifically studied. Cognitive-behavioral therapy may be helpful (option C). (p. 330)

14.8 Naltrexone has shown to be more effective than placebo for treating which of the following?

A. Intermittent explosive disorder.
B. Conduct disorder.
C. Kleptomania.
D. Pyromania.
E. Oppositional defiant disorder.

**The correct response is option C: Kleptomania.**

There are no standard treatments for kleptomania, but medication might be helpful in some patients (option C). Naltrexone has specifically been found more effective than placebo in a randomized controlled trial, but it requires careful monitoring and can cause nausea and vomiting. SSRI antidepressants also have been used to treat the disorder. **(p. 336)**

# —CHAPTER 15—

# Substance-Related and Addictive Disorders

15.1 A 48-year-old woman reports to her family physician that she has been drinking a bottle of wine two to three times per week for the past 3 years. She has not been successful in her attempts to cut back her drinking, and her drinking has led to conflicts with her family. She is occasionally late for work when she is hungover but has never had symptoms of alcohol withdrawal. Which of the following is the best diagnosis?

A. Alcohol use disorder.
B. Alcohol dependence.
C. Alcohol abuse.
D. Alcoholism.
E. Alcohol abuse disorder.

**The correct response is option A: Alcohol use disorder.**

Alcohol use disorder is the new DSM-5 disorder that merges the DSM-IV disorders of alcohol dependence and alcohol abuse (options B, C). Neither alcoholism nor alcohol abuse disorder (options D, E) is a DSM-5 diagnosis. Alcohol use disorder (option A) is further specified as mild, moderate, or severe, depending on the number of symptoms present. These diagnostic changes apply to all substance use disorders. Her disorder would qualify as mild, which is defined as the presence of two to three symptoms. **(pp. 346–349)**

15.2   Which neurotransmitter plays a key role in the development of all substance use disorders?

A. Serotonin.
B. Acetylcholine.
C. β-Endorphin.
D. Norepinephrine.
E. Dopamine.

**The correct response is option E: Dopamine.**

Research has begun to identify the neurobiological substrates of addiction. Dopamine pathways that form part of the central nervous system "reward system" have been identified in the ventral tegmental region of the forebrain and in the nucleus accumbens. All drugs of abuse appear to target the brain's reward system by flooding the circuit with dopamine (option E). **(p. 345)**

15.3   Which neurotransmitter plays a role specifically in the development of opioid use disorders?

A. Dopamine.
B. β-Endorphin.
C. Acetylcholine.
D. Serotonin.
E. Norepinephrine.

**The correct response is option B: β-Endorphin.**

Opioids activate μ receptors that release β-endorphins (option B), the chemical that is released when human beings engage in naturally rewarding activities (e.g., eating, sex). Dopamine (option A) modulates the reward system and is important in the development of all substance use disorders, but its importance is not specific to opioid use disorders. Acetylcholine (option C) has a major role in mediating memory. Serotonin (option D) has a role in modulating mood, anxiety, and aggression. Norepinephrine (option E) has a role in mediating the mood disorders. **(pp. 65–70, 345)**

15.4    A 17-year-old girl is referred for treatment of an alcohol use disorder. She drinks nearly every day (mostly beer and wine) and drinks to intoxication twice weekly. Her father drinks excessively, and the family receives government assistance. One reason she gives for her drinking is that her friends also drink, and it is hard for her not to go along with them. Which of the following variables is associated with a lesser risk for developing an alcohol use disorder?

A. Low socioeconomic status.
B. Susceptibility to peer influence.
C. Female sex.
D. Younger age.
E. Parental alcoholism.

**The correct response is option C: Female sex.**

The girl in the vignette unfortunately has many risk factors for an alcohol use disorder, which does not bode well for her future. That said, female sex is less likely to predispose to an alcohol use disorder than male sex (option C). Options A, B, D, and E are all factors associated with the development of an alcohol use disorder. **(pp. 344–346)**

15.5    How many positive responses on a CAGE test are needed to indicate that a person might have an alcohol use disorder?

A. One.
B. Two.
C. Three.
D. Four.
E. The CAGE test is not a good screening test for alcohol use disorders.

**The correct response is option A: One.**

Even one positive response or overly defensive answer on the CAGE test, a simple screen that can be used to assess the presence of an alcohol use disorder, can indicate problematic use (option A). A positive screen should be followed up with more detailed discussion. **(Table 15–2 [CAGE: screening test for an alcohol use disorder], p. 349; pp. 348–349)**

15.6  Which of the following develops as a late-stage consequence of an alcohol use disorder?

A. Decreased work productivity.
B. Moodiness or irritability.
C. Palmar erythema.
D. Rosacea.
E. Jaundice.

**The correct response is option E: Jaundice.**

Jaundice develops in the later stages of alcohol use disorder (option E) and indicates advanced liver disease. The symptoms in options A–D develop earlier in the course. **(p. 349)**

15.7  A 45-year-old man reports a 10-year history of heavy alcohol consumption to his family physician. He tells his physician that he is not as "sharp" as he used to be before he started drinking and that he has some mild difficulties with everyday memory tasks. He asks his doctor if these memory problems will be permanent. What is the best response?

A. "Even if you stop drinking, these memory problems are likely to be irreversible but not progressive."
B. "Even if you stop drinking, these memory problems are likely to be irreversible and progressive."
C. "If you stop drinking now, these memory problems may partially reverse."
D. "If you stop drinking now, your memory will likely fully recover."
E. None of the above.

**The correct response is option C: "If you stop drinking now, these memory problems may partially reverse."**

The physician can feel comfortable in sharing the good news: Neuropsychological testing of alcoholic persons generally reveals mild to moderate cognitive deficits that partially reverse with sobriety (option C). Chronic alcohol misuse also has been associated with enlarged cerebral ventricles and widened cortical sulci, effects that also may be partially reversible if the individual stops drinking. **(pp. 350–351)**

15.8    What percentage of motor vehicle deaths are related to alcohol use?

A. 10%.
B. 20%.
C. 30%.
D. 40%.
E. >50%.

**The correct response is option E: >50%.**

More than 50% of motor vehicle deaths are related to alcohol use (option E). **(p. 352)**

15.9    Which of the following are the last symptoms to develop during the course of severe alcohol withdrawal?

A. Delirium, fever, autonomic hyperarousal.
B. Auditory, visual, tactile hallucinations in the presence of a clear sensorium.
C. Seizures.
D. Anxiety, tremor, nausea.
E. Increased heart rate and blood pressure.

**The correct response is option A: Delirium, fever, autonomic hyperarousal.**

Alcohol withdrawal delirium, which includes fever and autonomic hyperarousal, develops 2–3 days after cessation or major reduction in drinking behavior (option A). The first symptoms to develop are anxiety, tremor, nausea, and increased heart rate and blood pressure (options D, E). These symptoms develop 12–18 hours after cessation or reduction in drinking. Seizures (option C) occur from 7 hours up to 2 days after cessation or reduction in drinking. Hallucinations (option B) can occur within 48 hours and can last for up to a week. **(p. 353)**

15.10 A psychiatrist is called to evaluate a 38-year-old man for admission to a psychiatric unit for alcohol detoxification and treatment of depression. He has been drinking large quantities of vodka daily for several months. He previously drank three to four beers nearly daily for almost 5 years. His last drink was 6 hours ago. He is currently pleasant and cooperative. He is fully oriented and in no distress. The psychiatrist asks the man if he has ever had delirium tremens (DTs). He responds, "Oh yeah, I've got the shakes right now," and he holds out his hands to show the psychiatrist his mild tremor. How shall the psychiatrist proceed?

A. Recommend admission to intensive care because DTs can be fatal.
B. Admit the patient to psychiatry for alcohol rehabilitation.
C. Administer chlordiazepoxide now.
D. Collect additional information such as if the man has ever had confusion and fever during withdrawal or had become agitated.
E. None of the above.

**The correct response is option D: Collect additional information such as if the man has ever had confusion and fever during withdrawal or had become agitated.**

Many patients (and physicians) are unaware of what constitutes an alcohol withdrawal delirium (the "DTs") and confuse tremors that develop during the earliest part of withdrawal with DTs. In these cases, the psychiatrist should collect additional information to determine if the patient has ever had an alcohol withdrawal delirium episode (option D). Patients at risk for severe withdrawal symptoms may require supportive care on a medical-surgical unit or an intensive care unit (option A). Disposition is best decided after information gathering is complete. Administering chlordiazepoxide (option C) or another benzodiazepine should be started, but this response option does not address the issue of patient disposition. Alcohol rehabilitation (option B) will be important later, but the man first needs to be withdrawn from alcohol while being medically monitored. **(pp. 352–355)**

15.11 Which medication used to treat alcohol dependence works by inhibiting aldehyde dehydrogenase?

A. Naltrexone.
B. Disulfiram.
C. Acamprosate.
D. Chlordiazepoxide.
E. Lorazepam.

**The correct response is option B: Disulfiram.**

Disulfiram inhibits aldehyde dehydrogenase, leading to the accumulation of acetaldehyde if the patient consumes alcohol, causing symptoms such as flushing, nausea, and vomiting (option B). Naltrexone (option A) is a μ-opioid antagonist and reduces cravings. Acamprosate (option C) is a glutamate receptor modulator that reduces cravings. Chlordiazepoxide and lorazepam (options D, E) are benzodiazepines that can be used to treat acute alcohol withdrawal. **(pp. 353, 356)**

15.12  A 20-year-old student sees his internist for anxiety symptoms. He reports that he has started worrying about everything since he started college about 2 years ago. He has trouble falling asleep and staying asleep nearly every night. His mood is mildly irritable, and he appears restless. He does not smoke, use alcohol, or use illicit drugs. He reports that he drinks eight or more cups of coffee daily to help him stay motivated when studying, with his last cup around 8:00–10:00 P.M. Which of the following is the most likely diagnosis?

A. Generalized anxiety disorder.
B. Bipolar I disorder.
C. Caffeine-induced anxiety disorder.
D. Panic disorder.
E. Insomnia disorder.

**The correct response is option C: Caffeine-induced anxiety disorder.**

Caffeine can cause or exacerbate anxiety disorders. Given this patient's excessive caffeine intake, caffeine-induced anxiety disorder is the best diagnosis (option C). Should he still complain of continued anxiety after significantly reducing his caffeine intake, generalized anxiety disorder (option A) would be a reasonable consideration. Irritability and insomnia in themselves are not sufficient to diagnose a manic episode associated with a bipolar disorder (option B). Panic attacks are acute spells of severe anxiety that last 15–20 minutes; therefore, panic disorder (option D) does not fit the pattern described in the vignette. Insomnia disorder (option E) would be a credible option if there was no history of excessive caffeine intake. **(pp. 142, 179, 187, 276, 357–358)**

15.13  Which of the following is *not* associated with cannabis use?

A. Increased risk of developing schizophrenia.
B. Increased risk of smoking cigarettes and abusing other drugs.
C. Tachycardia, dry mouth, and conjunctivitis during intoxication.
D. Flashbacks between periods of use.
E. Feeling that time has slowed and increased appetite during intoxication.

**The correct response is option D: Flashbacks between periods of use.**

Flashbacks between periods of use are associated with hallucinogens such as lysergic acid diethylamide (LSD) (option D). Options A–C and E are associated with cannabis use. **(p. 358)**

15.14  A 19-year-old man presents to the emergency department complaining of acute-onset severe anxiety, confusion, time expansion, and vivid visual hallucinations. He took LSD for the first time 3 hours ago and is very uncomfortable, but he is cooperative in interview. His pupils are dilated, and he has mild tachycardia. Reassurance fails to calm him down. Which of the following is the next best step in managing this case?

A. Give an antipsychotic.
B. Give a benzodiazepine.
C. Give clonidine.
D. Give naltrexone.
E. Refer the man to a substance use treatment program.

**The correct response is option B: Give a benzodiazepine.**

Benzodiazepines can be used to calm patients who develop severe anxiety secondary to hallucinogen intoxication when "talking them down" does not work (option B). Clonidine (option C) can be used to help patients through opioid withdrawal. Naltrexone (option D) is one alternative to help patients with an alcohol use disorder maintain abstinence. An antipsychotic (option A) may be necessary to calm a patient who develops agitation secondary to phencyclidine or stimulant use. Although this patient would benefit from some form of substance use disorder treatment, such a referral would not address his immediate report of anxiety secondary to acute hallucinogen intoxication (option E). **(pp. 359–360)**

15.15 A 30-year-old man requests help for an opioid abuse disorder. He has used large quantities of prescription narcotics obtained on the streets and will also inject heroin when it is available. He has tried to quit these drugs on his own several times without success. Which of the following is the best option to treat his opioid use disorder and reduce his risk of relapse and criminal activity?

A. Referral to Narcotics Anonymous.
B. Detoxification with clonidine followed by outpatient counseling.
C. Referral to a methadone or buprenorphine maintenance program following detoxification.
D. Prescribing naltrexone.
E. Detoxification with clonidine followed by referral to an intensive outpatient program.

**The correct response is option C: Referral to a methadone or buprenorphine maintenance program following detoxification.**

Maintenance programs that provide methadone or buprenorphine have been shown to reduce risk of relapse, depression, and criminal activity and to improve the functional status of patients with opioid use disorders. These programs typically provide counseling services in addition to the medication following detoxification. The other response options (A, B, E) could each be useful, but option C is the most appropriate choice for this patient. Naltrexone (option D) has no role in the treatment of opioid use disorders. **(pp. 362–363, 370)**

15.16 A 26-year-old woman comes to your office seeking help for anxiety and panic attacks. She was last seen by your colleague a week ago, but she reports that she has lost her prescription for alprazolam. She asks you to write a new prescription for alprazolam 3 mg four times daily. She reports that nothing else works and that she has allergies to the selective serotonin reuptake inhibitors. Which of the following is *not* a valid reason to have serious concerns about prescribing alprazolam to this patient?

A. Concern about doctor-shopping behavior.
B. Report that "nothing else works."
C. Report of severe allergies to other medications commonly used to treat anxiety.
D. Report of a lost prescription.
E. Lethality of benzodiazepines in overdose.

**The correct response is option E: Lethality of benzodiazepines in overdose.**

Benzodiazepines have a very high therapeutic window and are not often lethal in overdose (option E). Options A–D all constitute very good reasons to have serious concerns about prescribing this patient a benzodiazepine. **(pp. 364–365)**

15.17  A 23-year-old man with no psychiatric history is brought to the emergency department by the police for agitated and disorganized behavior. He is paranoid and believes that the government is sending him messages through a microchip that was implanted in one of his teeth. He has not slept for 3 days. He is distractible in interview but otherwise oriented. A urine drug screen is positive for amphetamine. He is otherwise medically stable and is admitted to the psychiatry unit. What is the best course of treatment for this patient's psychotic symptoms?

A. Supportive care and possibly short-term use of antipsychotic.
B. Antipsychotic therapy for 6 months.
C. Cognitive-behavioral psychotherapy.
D. Imipramine.
E. Lithium.

**The correct response is option A: Supportive care and possibly short-term use of antipsychotic.**

Stimulant-induced psychoses generally resolve with sobriety; therefore, supportive care and a short-term antipsychotic is the best course of treatment (option A). Long-term use of an antipsychotic (option B) is not necessary. Antidepressants (option D) and psychotherapy (option C) will not treat the psychosis. The patient's insomnia and psychotic symptoms are more likely due to methamphetamine use than bipolar I disorder given the urine drug screen results; therefore, use of lithium (option E) is not indicated. **(p. 366)**

15.18 Your patient tells you that he plans to stop smoking cigarettes because he realizes that it constitutes a major health hazard. He asks for your advice about how to quit successfully. Which of the following is most likely to help your patient quit smoking?

A. Bupropion.
B. Quitting "cold turkey."
C. Nicotine gum.
D. Varenicline.
E. A combination of nicotine gum and varenicline.

**The correct response is option E: A combination of nicotine gum and varenicline.**

Options A, C, and D are effective, but combined treatment, either nicotine gum or a transdermal patch and bupropion or varenicline, likely leads to the best outcome (option E). Quitting "cold turkey" (option B) will lead to nicotine withdrawal, usually starting 1 hour after the last cigarette is smoked. Symptoms include nicotine craving, irritability, anxiety, and restlessness. Nicotine replacement therapy, bupropion, and varenicline all help to mitigate these symptoms. **(pp. 367–368)**

15.19 What form of therapy for substance use disorders rewards patients for appropriate behavior (e.g., giving patients who submit clean urine samples vouchers that can be exchanged for retail goods and services)?

A. Contingency management.
B. Motivational interviewing.
C. Cognitive-behavioral therapy.
D. Behavioral activation.
E. Twelve-step program.

**The correct response is option A: Contingency management.**

Contingency management rewards appropriate behavior with material goods (option A). Motivational interviewing (option B) helps patients to make their own argument for change. Cognitive-behavioral therapy (option C) addresses negative automatic thoughts and core beliefs and explores how thoughts, feelings, and behaviors relate. Behavioral activation (option D), a component of cognitive therapy, seeks to reengage depressed patients in their usual activities. Twelve-step programs (option E) such as Alcoholics Anonymous provide regular supportive community meetings to help patients maintain and achieve abstinence from alcohol and other substances of abuse. **(pp. 355, 369–370, 453)**

15.20 Which of the following treatments has a role in treating gambling disorder?

A. Gamblers Anonymous.
B. Naltrexone.
C. Motivational interviewing.
D. Cognitive-behavioral therapy.
E. All the above.

**The correct response is option E: All the above.**

Although there is no standard treatment for gambling disorder, all the treatments listed have a role (option E). Gamblers Anonymous (option A) is a self-help group patterned after Alcoholics Anonymous and provides support and encouragement to persons in recovery from gambling disorder. Naltrexone (option B) has been shown in clinical trials to reduce gambling urges. Motivational interviewing and cognitive-behavioral therapy (options C, D) are often combined in the psychotherapeutic treatment of gambling disorder. **(p. 372)**

# CHAPTER 16

# Neurocognitive Disorders

16.1    Which of the following is a neurocognitive disorder new to DSM-5?

A. Social cognitive disorder.
B. Alzheimer's dementia.
C. Major cognitive impairment disorder.
D. Mild neurocognitive disorder.
E. Dementia disorder.

**The correct response is option D: Mild neurocognitive disorder.**

DSM-5 transformed the classification of the neurocognitive disorders by introducing two new categories—major neurocognitive disorder and mild neurocognitive disorder (option D)—that are distinguished based on severity. Diagnostic criteria are provided for each disorder followed by criteria for specific etiological subtypes (e.g., major neurocognitive disorder due to Alzheimer's disease). Mild neurocognitive disorder is an important new category because it acknowledges less severe levels of impairment that can also be a focus of care. Options A–C and E are not DSM-5 diagnoses. **(pp. 375–376, 387–389)**

16.2    Processing speed is a part of which cognitive domain?

A. Social cognition.
B. Complex attention.
C. Learning and memory.
D. Executive function.
E. Language.

The correct response is option B: Complex attention.

The criteria for major and mild neurocognitive disorders are based on six defined key cognitive domains. They are complex attention, executive function (option D), learning and memory (option C), language (option E), perceptual motor ability, and social cognition (option A). Complex attention encompasses sustained attention, divided attention, selective attention, and processing speed (option B). **(pp. 376–377)**

16.3   Which of the following is *not* a risk factor for delirium?

A. Use of narcotics.
B. Recent surgery.
C. Older age.
D. Preexisting depression.
E. Systemic infection.

**The correct response is option D: Preexisting depression.**

Elderly patients are at high risk for delirium (option C), especially those older than 80 years. Additional risk factors include a preexisting dementia, recent surgery (option B), bone fractures, systemic infections (option E), and recent use of narcotics (option A) or antipsychotics. Preexisting depression is not a known risk factor for delirium (option D). **(p. 378)**

16.4   Which of the following is *least* consistent with delirium?

A. Fluctuation in mental status throughout the day.
B. Disturbance of memory.
C. Occurrence in a hospitalized patient receiving narcotics.
D. Patient reports of visual and tactile hallucinations.
E. Insidious onset.

**The correct response is option E: Insidious onset.**

Delirium typically has an acute onset over a few days rather than an insidious onset over weeks to months (option E). Visual and tactile hallucinations (option D) are common in delirium, although they are not required for the diagnosis. Narcotics (option C) can induce delirium and should be avoided. Fluctuations in mental status throughout the day and memory disturbance (options A, B) are features of delirium. **(pp. 377–378)**

16.5 In which of the following patients are benzodiazepines *least* likely to worsen his or her delirium?

A. A highly agitated 25-year-old man hospitalized for 2 weeks for encephalopathy.
B. A calm 32-year-old woman hospitalized for 1 week for pneumonia.
C. A 65-year-old man with a severe alcohol use disorder hospitalized for the past 3 days recovering from abdominal surgery.
D. An agitated 75-year-old woman with sepsis who reports vivid visual hallucinations.
E. Any patient with delirium.

**The correct response is option C: A 65-year-old man with a severe alcohol use disorder hospitalized for the past 3 days recovering from abdominal surgery.**

A benzodiazepine may be helpful for the surgical patient with an alcohol use disorder because it is likely that this patient's delirium is due to alcohol withdrawal (option C). In patients who do not have alcohol withdrawal, benzodiazepines should be avoided because they can worsen delirium. **(pp. 380–381)**

16.6 Which of the following distinguishes a major and mild neurocognitive disorder?

A. Decline in memory from baseline.
B. Presence of attentional difficulties.
C. Presence of impairment on neuropsychological assessment.
D. Acute onset over days.
E. Impairment in ability to live independently.

**The correct response is option E: Impairment in ability to live independently.**

Major neurocognitive disorder causes an impairment in a person's ability to live independently, whereas a mild neurocognitive disorder does not (option E). Acute onset over days is more characteristic of a delirium (option D). Both major and mild neurocognitive disorders show some degree of impairment on neuropsychological assessment (option C), but the degree of impairment will be greater for major neurocognitive disorders. Patients with either major or mild neurocognitive disorders can present with memory impairment (option A) or attentional difficulties (option B). **(pp. 381–387)**

16.7    What percentage of patients with a major neurocognitive disorder due to Alzheimer's disease develop psychotic symptoms such as hallucinations and delusions as their illness progresses?

    A.  1%.
    B.  5%.
    C.  10%.
    D.  25%.
    E.  50%.

**The correct response is option E: 50%.**

About half of patients with major neurocognitive disorder due to Alzheimer's disease develop hallucinations and delusions (option E). **(p. 384)**

16.8    A 67-year-old retired accountant presents to his family physician accompanied by his wife. His wife reports that he has been having progressive difficulty remembering appointments and important dates over the past 2 years, and she no longer allows him to drive. There are no current safety concerns at home. Brief cognitive assessment shows that he has impaired short-term recall and difficulty drawing a clock. What is the next best step in management of this case?

    A.  Referral to a skilled nursing facility.
    B.  Medical workup.
    C.  Neuropsychological assessment.
    D.  Start donepezil.
    E.  Referral to a psychiatrist to confirm diagnosis of a neurocognitive disorder.

**The correct response is option B: Medical workup.**

Patients who have a suspected neurocognitive disorder should have a medical workup to look for potential reversible causes of neurocognitive disorder (option B). Suggested studies include a complete blood count; liver, thyroid, and renal function tests; serologic tests for syphilis and HIV; urinalysis; electrocardiogram; and chest X-ray. Serum electrolytes, serum glucose, and vitamin $B_{12}$ and folate levels should be measured. Brain imaging should be obtained; an electroencephalogram (EEG) may be helpful as well if there is a concern for seizure activity. **(pp. 384–386)**

16.9 Which test can distinguish major neurocognitive disorder due to Alzheimer's disease from other neurocognitive disorders?

A. Magnetic resonance imaging (MRI).
B. Functional MRI.
C. Fluorodeoxyglucose positron emission tomography (PET).
D. Lumbar puncture.
E. Alzheimer's disease can only be confirmed on autopsy.

**The correct response is option C: Fluorodeoxyglucose positron emission tomography (PET).**

Fluorodeoxyglucose PET imaging can distinguish major neurocognitive disorder due to Alzheimer's disease from other neurocognitive disorders (option C). It will show characteristic parietal and temporal hypometabolism. Options A, B, and D may be useful in a medical workup of dementia. An autopsy (option E) is the definitive test for Alzheimer's disease but not in the living patient! **(p. 386)**

16.10 A 59-year-old woman is brought to her family physician accompanied by her spouse. She has had worsening of short-term memory and progressive apathy over the past month. She also reports low mood, insomnia, and low appetite, and she has lost 10 pounds since the symptoms began. She answers "I don't know" to many basic questions on a brief cognitive assessment. Which of the following medications would be of most benefit to this patient?

A. Donepezil.
B. Tacrine.
C. Sertraline.
D. Aripiprazole.
E. Memantine.

**The correct response is option C: Sertraline.**

In addition to memory disturbance, this patient endorses symptoms consistent with a major depressive episode. This is the *dementia syndrome of depression* (pseudodementia), but it is not a DSM-5 diagnosis. In these cases, an antidepressant such as sertraline will treat the depression, thereby improving cognition as the depression lifts (option C). However, the person with pseudodementia is at risk for developing a neurocognitive disorder in the future. **(p. 387)**

16.11  Which of the following is most specific for Alzheimer's disease?

A. Neurofibrillary tangles.
B. β-Amyloid plaques.
C. Hyperphosphorylated tau protein.
D. Apolipoprotein E polymorphism.
E. All the above are equally specific changes.

**The correct response is option B: β-Amyloid plaques.**

β-Amyloid plaques in the brain are a characteristic histopathological change in Alzheimer's disease (option B). Neurofibrillary tangles (option A), which are made up of hyperphosphorylated tau proteins (option C), are found in other neurodegenerative diseases in addition to Alzheimer's disease. Apolipoprotein E polymorphisms (option D) influence an individual's risk of developing Alzheimer's disease. **(p. 390)**

16.12  Primary progressive aphasia and a behavioral-variant subtype occur in which neurocognitive disorder?

A. Alzheimer's disease.
B. Frontotemporal neurocognitive disorder.
C. Neurocognitive disorder with Lewy bodies.
D. Vascular neurocognitive disorder.
E. None of the above.

**The correct response is option B: Frontotemporal neurocognitive disorder.**

Frontotemporal neurocognitive disorder (formerly Pick's disease) has a behavioral-variant subtype that presents with varying degrees of apathy or disinhibition (option B). Patients might lose interest in socialization, self-care, and personal responsibilities, or display socially inappropriate behaviors. The language-variant subtype presents with primary progressive aphasia with gradual onset. **(pp. 390–391)**

16.13 Which neurocognitive disorder is sometimes associated with rapid eye movement (REM) sleep behavior disorder?

A. Alzheimer's disease.
B. Frontotemporal neurocognitive disorder.
C. Neurocognitive disorder with Lewy bodies.
D. Vascular neurocognitive disorder.
E. None of the above.

**The correct response is option C: Neurocognitive disorder with Lewy bodies.**

Neurocognitive disorder with Lewy bodies (option C) is associated with REM sleep behavior disorder. Options A, B, and D do not have this association. **(pp. 387–392)**

16.14 A 67-year-old man is brought in by his family to see his family physician. They are concerned because he has had progressive difficulty keeping up with daily chores at home and is more irritable than usual. He tells the physician that he wouldn't be so irritable if his wife hadn't moved so many of her friends into the house. His wife reports that they live alone, and he seems to see people who aren't there. The patient is oriented and attends to the interview without difficulty. The physician notices that the patient has a shuffling gait. Which of the following is the most likely diagnosis?

A. Alzheimer's disease.
B. Frontotemporal neurocognitive disorder.
C. Neurocognitive disorder with Lewy bodies.
D. Vascular neurocognitive disorder.
E. Dementia.

**The correct response is option C: Neurocognitive disorder with Lewy bodies.**

Neurocognitive disorder with Lewy bodies is associated with visual hallucinations. The first cognitive changes noted tend to be problems with executive function, complex attention, and subtle personality changes (option C). Hallucinations can occur in other neurocognitive disorders such as Alzheimer's disease (option A), but they usually occur later in the disease process. Parkinsonian features may begin after the onset of cognitive decline. A person with frontotemporal neurocognitive disorder (option B) is likely to present with apathy or disinhibition. Vascular neurocognitive disorder (option D) is common, but a person with this disorder is likely to present with focal neurological deficits. Dementia (option E) is a generic term that in DSM-5 has been replaced by the term *neurocognitive disorder*. **(pp. 387–392)**

16.15 A rapid, progressive stepwise cognitive decline suggests which neurocognitive disorder?

A. Alzheimer's disease.
B. Frontotemporal neurocognitive disorder.
C. Neurocognitive disorder with Lewy bodies.
D. Vascular neurocognitive disorder.
E. Delirium.

**The correct response is option D: Vascular neurocognitive disorder.**

Vascular neurocognitive disorder will often show a stepwise decline because the cognitive deficits are secondary to ischemic events (option D). Delirium (option E) has an acute onset of impairment in attention and altered sensorium, and it is often reversible with treatment of the underlying cause. Alzheimer's disease, frontotemporal neurocognitive disorder, and neurocognitive disorder with Lewy bodies (options A–C) present with an insidious, gradual decline rather than stepwise decline. **(pp. 377–380, 387–392)**

16.16 A 25-year-old man recently diagnosed with an HIV infection sees his internist to address some concerns. He has read about "HIV dementia," and he asks his physician about his risk of developing this complication. What is the most accurate response?

A. "It's a rare complication, so your risk is low."
B. "You have a high risk of developing this condition at some point."

C. "We can't determine this at the present."
D. "There's a fair chance you may eventually develop some mild cognitive problems, but your risk of developing severe cognitive problems is low."
E. None of the above.

**The correct response is option D: "There's a fair chance you may eventually develop some mild cognitive problems, but your risk of developing severe cognitive problems is low."**

Up to 25% of patients with HIV will develop a mild neurocognitive disorder, but the chances of developing a major neurocognitive disorder secondary to HIV are less than 5% (option D). **(p. 393)**

16.17 Which of the following findings is characteristic of Creutzfeldt-Jakob disease?

A. Triphasic complexes on EEG.
B. Diffuse slowing on EEG.
C. Hypocretin deficiency.
D. Degeneration of the mamillary bodies.
E. Hypometabolism of parietal and temporal areas on PET scan.

**The correct response is option A: Triphasic complexes on EEG.**

Triphasic complexes on EEG are characteristic of Creutzfeldt-Jakob disease (option A), although a new variant that lacks this finding has been identified. Diffuse slowing on EEG (option B) suggests delirium. Hypocretin deficiency (option C) suggests the sleep disorder narcolepsy. Degeneration of the mamillary bodies (option D) occurs in Wernicke-Korsakoff syndrome. Hypometabolism of parietal and temporal areas on PET scan (option E) is characteristic of Alzheimer's disease. **(pp. 281, 350, 380, 386, 393–394)**

16.18 Dementia, gait disturbance, and urinary incontinence are the classic triad of which medical condition that can cause a neurocognitive disorder?

A. Pellagra.
B. Prion disease.
C. Subdural hematoma.

D. Alcohol use.

E. Normal-pressure hydrocephalus.

**The correct response is option E: Normal-pressure hydrocephalus.**

Normal-pressure hydrocephalus is classically associated with cognitive decline, gait disturbance, and urinary incontinence (option E). Long-term, heavy alcohol use (option D) can cause some cognitive decline and some cerebellar degeneration, which may result in some degree of ataxia. Subdural hematoma (option C) and pellagra (option A) can cause cognitive disorder, but the forms that these cognitive disorders take do not have established characteristic features. Prion disease (option B) causes a rapidly progressive, fatal cognitive decline that is associated with myoclonus and akinetic mutism. **(pp. 350, 393, 395–396)**

16.19 Which of the following medications is an appropriate choice to help with nighttime agitation, or "sundowning," in patients with neurocognitive disorders?

A. Lithium.

B. Carbamazepine.

C. Divalproex.

D. Trazodone.

E. Chlorpromazine.

**The correct response is option D: Trazodone.**

A bedtime dose of trazodone can help with sundowning in patients with neurocognitive disorders (option D). Chlorpromazine (option E) and other low-potency, first-generation antipsychotics should be avoided because their anticholinergic activity can worsen cognition. Lithium, carbamazepine, and divalproex (options A–C) have no clear role in treating the behavioral complications of neurocognitive disorders. **(p. 397)**

16.20 Which of the following cognitive-enhancing drugs works on *N*-methyl-D-aspartate (NMDA) receptors?

A. Donepezil.

B. Tacrine.

C. Memantine.
D. Rivastigmine.
E. Galantamine.

**The correct response is option C: Memantine.**

Memantine blocks NMDA receptors that normally bind gluta-mate (option C). The agents in options A, B, D, and E are cholin-esterase inhibitors. **(p. 396)**

16.21 Why has the U.S. Food and Drug Administration (FDA) issued a black box warning about the use of second-generation antipsy-chotics in elderly patients with neurocognitive disorders?

A. They are associated with an increased rate of cognitive de-cline.
B. They are associated with severe gastrointestinal side effects.
C. They are associated with an increased risk of mortality.
D. Liver enzymes must be monitored regularly.
E. They have no benefit for managing disruptive behaviors in patients with neurocognitive disorders.

**The correct response is option C: They are associated with an increased risk of mortality.**

The FDA issued a warning about the use of second-generation antipsychotics in elderly patients with neurocognitive disorders because of an increased risk of mortality (option C). These agents have been used off-label to help control disruptive behaviors and psychosis (option E). Cholinesterase inhibitors can cause gastro-intestinal symptoms, but the symptoms are usually not severe and are not subject to a black box warning (option D). Liver en-zymes must be monitored with use of the cholinesterase inhibi-tor tacrine (option D), which is not in common use. There is no evidence that second-generation antipsychotics are associated with cognitive decline (option A). **(pp. 396–398)**

# —CHAPTER 17—

# Personality Disorders

17.1 Which was the first DSM to include disturbances of personality?

A. DSM-I.
B. DSM-II.
C. DSM-III.
D. DSM-IV.
E. DSM-5.

**The correct response is option A: DSM-I.**

Published in 1952, DSM-I included seven types of personality disturbance (option A), and personality disorders have been a part of each subsequent edition. The disorders are unchanged from DSM-IV to DSM-5. **(p. 401)**

17.2 Which of the following is *not* true of the general criteria of a personality disorder?

A. The behavior is consistent with the individual's cultural expectations.
B. It is stable over time with onset in adolescence or early adulthood.
C. The disorder leads to distress or impairment.
D. The disorder is not limited to episodes of illness.
E. All the above are part of the general criteria of a personality disorder.

**The correct response is option A: The behavior is consistent with the individual's cultural expectations.**

Personality disorders represent an enduring pattern of inner experience and behavior that deviates markedly from the expectations of an individual's culture (option A). Options B–D are part of the general criteria of a personality disorder. **(pp. 401–402)**

17.3   A patient has long-standing discrete episodes of mania and depression dating to late adolescence. During manic episodes, he displays elevated mood, decreased sleep, pressured speech, and flight of ideas. The episodes typically result in psychiatric hospitalization. During the manic episodes, he engages in antisocial behavior, including committing assaults and writing bad checks. He is a quiet, law-abiding citizen between episodes of mania. Which of the following is the most likely diagnosis?

A. Antisocial personality disorder.
B. Bipolar I disorder.
C. Personality disorder due to bipolar I disorder.
D. Bipolar I disorder plus antisocial personality disorder.
E. None of the above.

**The correct response is option B: Bipolar I disorder.**

This patient cannot be diagnosed with antisocial personality disorder (option A) because his antisocial behavior is limited to episodes of mania. For that reason, bipolar I disorder plus antisocial personality disorder (option D) is also inappropriate. Per the general criteria of a personality disorder, deviant behavior cannot be limited to discrete episodes of illness. Personality disorder due to bipolar I disorder (option C) is not a DSM-5 diagnosis. **(pp. 142–144, 401–402, 412–414)**

17.4   A patient has long-standing discrete episodes of mania and depression dating back to late adolescence. During the manic episodes, he has elevated mood, decreased sleep, pressured speech, and flight of ideas that typically result in psychiatric hospitalization. He gets into more legal trouble than usual during these periods, but even during periods of euthymia, he tends to engage in illegal activities such as shoplifting and burglary. He has done so since early adolescence, and he does not show any remorse for these actions. Which of the following is the most likely diagnosis?

A. Antisocial personality disorder.
B. Bipolar I disorder.

C. Personality disorder due to bipolar I disorder.

D. Bipolar I disorder plus antisocial personality disorder.

E. None of the above.

**The correct response is option D: Bipolar I disorder plus antisocial personality disorder.**

In contrast to the patient in question 17.3, this patient has a long-standing pattern of antisocial behavior that is not limited to episodes of his illness. Therefore, it is most appropriate to diagnose him with both antisocial personality disorder and bipolar I disorder (option D). Personality disorder secondary to bipolar I disorder (option C) is not a DSM-5 diagnosis. Bipolar I disorder (option B) and antisocial personality disorder (option A) are inappropriate because they do not account for the combination of disorders seen in this man. **(pp. 142–144, 401–402, 412–414)**

17.5 Which of the following personality disorders is *not* a Cluster C personality disorder?

A. Avoidant personality disorder.

B. Obsessive-compulsive personality disorder.

C. Histrionic personality disorder.

D. Dependent personality disorder.

E. All the above are Cluster C personality disorders.

**The correct response is option C: Histrionic personality disorder.**

The Cluster C personality disorders are avoidant, obsessive-compulsive, and dependent personality disorders (options A, B, D). Histrionic personality disorder (option C) is a Cluster B personality disorder. Cluster B ("dramatic cluster") personality disorders share dramatic, emotional, and erratic characteristics. **(Table 17–1 [DSM-5 personality disorders], p. 402)**

17.6 Which of the following does *not* represent a major personality trait according to personality theorists who favor a dimensional perspective?

A. Extraversion.

B. Agreeableness.

C. Openness to experience.

D. Genuineness.

E. Neuroticism.

**The correct response is option D: Genuineness.**

The best-known dimensional personality model was developed by psychologists Paul Costa and Robert McCrae and is known as the five-factor model. The traits outlined by the model include extraversion, agreeableness (options A, B), conscientiousness (not genuineness [option D]), openness to experience, and neuroticism (options C, E). **(p. 403)**

17.7 Which of the following personality disorders occurs about equally in men and women?

A. Antisocial personality disorder.

B. Borderline personality disorder.

C. Histrionic personality disorder.

D. Dependent personality disorder.

E. Schizotypal personality disorder.

**The correct response is option E: Schizotypal personality disorder.**

Schizotypal personality disorder (option E) is equally common in men and women. Antisocial personality disorder is more common in men (option A). Borderline, histrionic, and dependent personality disorders (options B–D) are more common in women. **(p. 403)**

17.8 Which of the following is the only personality disorder with an age requirement and a requirement that certain childhood behaviors have continuity with adult traits?

A. Antisocial personality disorder.

B. Borderline personality disorder.

C. Avoidant personality disorder.

D. Dependent personality disorder.

E. Schizotypal personality disorder.

**The correct response is option A: Antisocial personality disorder.**

Antisocial personality disorder is not diagnosed before age 18 years. The criteria require evidence of conduct disorder (option A) before age 15 years. DSM-5 requires that the maladaptive personality features be present for at least 1 year if a personality disorder is diagnosed before 18 years. The other personality disorders (options B–E) do not have an age requirement. Although no other personality disorder has child or adolescent criteria, research suggests that behavioral precursors such as affective lability or impulsivity can sometimes be traced back to childhood. Personality pathology in childhood or adolescence is predictive of adult maladjustment and the later development of a personality disorder. **(pp. 403, 412–414)**

17.9 Does the diagnosis of a personality disorder tend to be stable over time?

A. Most personality disorders are diagnostically stable throughout life, but the severity may diminish with age.
B. Most personality disorders are diagnostically stable, and symptom severity is stable.
C. Severity of personality disorders diminishes, and many people will make a full psychosocial recovery.
D. Severity of personality disorders diminishes, but many people will still have some degree of interpersonal dysfunction.
E. None of the above.

**The correct response is option D: Severity of personality disorders diminishes, but many people will still have some degree of interpersonal dysfunction.**

The severity of personality disorders tends to diminish with advancing age, and many patients will no longer meet full criteria for a given disorder. Most will continue to have some degree of impairment in important life domains (option D). **(p. 404)**

17.10 Which of the following has *not* been shown to contribute to the risk of developing a personality disorder?

A. Being a victim of child abuse.
B. Witnessing domestic violence in the home.
C. Parental divorce or separation.
D. Parental absence.
E. Arrested psychosexual development.

**The correct response is option E: Arrested psychosexual development.**

Psychoanalysts have postulated that maladaptive personality traits arise from arrested psychosexual development (option E), but there is no evidence to support this view. Options A–D have all been shown to contribute to the risk of developing a personality disorder. **(pp. 404–405)**

17.11 Which of the following personality disorders is associated with impaired smooth pursuit eye movement, impaired performance on tests of executive function, and increased ventricular-brain ratio on computed tomography?

A. Antisocial personality disorder.
B. Borderline personality disorder.
C. Schizotypal personality disorder.
D. Schizoid personality disorder.
E. Avoidant personality disorder.

**The correct response is option C: Schizotypal personality disorder.**

Schizotypal personality disorder, long considered to fall within a spectrum of disorders related to schizophrenia, is associated with impaired smooth pursuit eye movement, impaired performance on tests of executive function, and increased ventricular-brain ratio on computed tomography (option C). **(p. 405)**

17.12 Which of the following personality disorders is associated with low resting pulse, low skin conductance, and increased amplitude on event-related potentials?

A. Antisocial personality disorder.
B. Borderline personality disorder.
C. Schizotypal personality disorder.
D. Schizoid personality disorder.
E. Avoidant personality disorder.

**The correct response is option A: Antisocial personality disorder.**

Antisocial personality disorder is associated with low resting pulse, low skin conductance, and increased amplitude on event-related potentials (option A). These findings suggest to some that antisocial persons are chronically underaroused and seek out potentially risky situations to raise their arousal to more optimal levels. Options B–E are not associated with these findings. **(p. 405)**

17.13 A 27-year-old software engineer seeks psychiatric treatment for anxiety. He has lived alone all his adult life. Outside of work, he has no social contacts apart from a weekly telephone call to his mother. He spends most of his free time playing video games, and he expresses little interest in developing more social relationships or having a romantic relationship. He does not endorse any symptoms of major depression or psychosis. He is very stiff and formal in interview and displays little emotion. Which of the following is the most likely diagnosis?

A. Avoidant personality disorder.
B. Schizotypal personality disorder.
C. Schizoid personality disorder.
D. Autism spectrum disorder.
E. Antisocial personality disorder.

**The correct response is option C: Schizoid personality disorder.**

Patients with schizoid personality disorder have a profound defect in the ability to form personal relationships and to respond to others in a meaningful way (option C). Patients with avoidant personality disorder (option A) typically desire social contact, but their anxiety interferes with developing relationships in the absence of significant reassurance. Patients with schizotypal personality disorder (option B) tend to have few relationships but are odd and eccentric with unusual thinking and speech. Although autism spectrum disorder (option D) is not a bad choice in that people with these disorders often have few relationships, they also have significant impairments in social communication and restricted and repetitive patterns of behavior, which the patient in the vignette does not have. Patients with antisocial personality disorder (option E) are antisocial in the sense that they do not have respect for the rights of others, not because of impaired social skills. **(pp. 93–99, 409–413, 419)**

17.14 You see a 33-year-old unemployed man in the outpatient clinic. He reports that he would like your assistance in getting disability for "anxiety." He says that for as long as he recalls, he has felt uncomfortable in social situations because he fears that other people will not understand him. He has never married and has no children. He has trouble maintaining employment because of anxiety. He sometimes thinks that magazine articles have special messages for him and may see shadows that look like people or animals. He has been trying to learn how to communicate telepathically by studying a "new age" book purchased on the Internet but has not been successful. He denies any history of auditory hallucinations and does not appear to have delusions. Which of the following is the most likely diagnosis?

A. Schizophrenia.
B. Schizotypal personality disorder.
C. Avoidant personality disorder.
D. Schizoid personality disorder.
E. Schizoaffective disorder.

**The correct response is option B: Schizotypal personality disorder.**

The man in the vignette best meets the spirit of schizotypal personality disorder (option B). Such patients are odd and eccentric and typically have unusual thinking and speech. Patients with schizoid personality disorder (option D) have a profound defect in the ability to form personal relationships and to respond to others in a meaningful way, but also tend not to be otherwise strange or eccentric. Patients with schizophrenia or schizoaffective disorder (options A, E) have frank delusions and hallucinations, in contrast to the nonpsychotic symptoms of patients with schizotypal personality disorder. Patients with avoidant personality disorder (option C) have difficulty forming relationships because of severe social anxiety. **(pp. 122–140, 409–412, 419)**

17.15 Which of the following is *not* a trait of histrionic personality disorder?

A. Unease in situations in which one is not the center of attention.
B. Inappropriate sexually seductive or provocative behavior.
C. Rapidly shifting and shallow expression of emotions.
D. Transient, stress-related paranoid ideation or severe dissociative symptoms.
E. Self-dramatization, theatricality, and exaggerated expression of emotion.

**The correct response is option D: Transient, stress-related paranoid ideation or severe dissociative symptoms.**

Transient, stress-related paranoid ideation or severe dissociative symptoms is a trait of borderline personality disorder (option D). Options A–C and E represent traits of histrionic personality disorder. **(pp. 416–417)**

17.16 A 26-year-old woman comes to your clinic to establish care for her mood swings that other psychiatrists have diagnosed as "bipolar disorder." She has persistent depression and severe mood swings, but she has never had a period of decreased sleep, pressured speech, or disinhibition that lasted for several days. She uses a razor blade to make small cuts on her forearms when anxious or upset but denies that she does this to kill herself. She has had several psychiatric hospitalizations for suicidal ideation, and she has overdosed multiple times. She endorses a deep fear that her loved ones will abandon her, and she has chronic feelings of emptiness. After your interview, she says that she thinks you are the best doctor she has ever had and that she has great confidence in your abilities. She speaks very poorly of her previous psychiatrist. Which of the following is the most likely diagnosis?

A. Bipolar II disorder.
B. Histrionic personality disorder.
C. Borderline personality disorder.
D. Dependent personality disorder.
E. Schizotypal personality disorder.

**The correct response is option C: Borderline personality disorder.**

Patients with borderline personality disorder experience mood instability and disturbed interpersonal relationships; fears of abandonment are common (option C). Patients with bipolar II disorder (option A) have discrete episodes of hypomania and depression. Histrionic personality disorder (option B) is characterized by attention-seeking behavior and shallow affect but not self-harm or mood instability. Patients with dependent personality disorder (option D) are overly reliant on others to meet their needs. Patients with schizotypal personality disorder (option E) have odd speech and thinking but do not report mood instability and are not chronically suicidal. **(pp. 146, 411, 414–416, 420)**

17.17 Which of the following is *not* a recommended treatment for borderline personality disorder?

    A. Dialectical behavior therapy.
    B. Benzodiazepines for accompanying anxiety.
    C. Systems Training for Emotional Predictability and Problem Solving (STEPPS).
    D. Antipsychotic medications for perceptual distortions and anger dyscontrol.
    E. Selective serotonin reuptake inhibitors (SSRIs) for depression.

**The correct response is option B: Benzodiazepines for accompanying anxiety.**

There are no standard treatments for borderline personality disorder, but several evidence-based group treatment programs appear to reduce the overall severity of the disorder. These include dialectical behavior therapy (option A) and STEPPS (option C). No medications are U.S. Food and Drug Administration approved to treat *any* personality disorder, including borderline personality disorder. Depressed patients with borderline personality disorder may benefit from antidepressants such as SSRIs (option E), whereas many symptoms of borderline personality disorder might improve with antipsychotics (option D). Benzodiazepines (option B) should be avoided because of their abuse potential and tendency to cause behavioral disinhibition. **(pp. 415–416)**

17.18 A 40-year-old business executive seeks treatment for depression. She reports being upset since a colleague was given a promotion that she feels was rightfully hers. Her long-term goal is to become the CEO of a major global corporation. During the session, she questions the therapist's credentials, and at one point she accuses the therapist of being envious of her superior social status. She does not return after the first session and later tells an acquaintance that it was because the therapist didn't give her the admiration that she deserves. Which of the following is the most likely diagnosis?

    A. Antisocial personality disorder.
    B. Borderline personality disorder.
    C. Narcissistic personality disorder.
    D. Dependent personality disorder.
    E. Histrionic personality disorder.

**The correct response is option C: Narcissistic personality disorder.**

Narcissistic personality disorder is characterized by exaggerated sense of self-importance and lack of empathy (option C). The other response options are not plausible, although many narcissistic persons will have symptoms consistent with some of the other personality disorders. Patients with dependent personality disorder (option D) are overly reliant on others to meet their needs. Histrionic personality disorder (option E) is characterized by attention-seeking behavior and shallow affect. Patients with borderline personality disorder (option B) have mood instability, fear of abandonment, and disturbed interpersonal relationships. Patients with antisocial personality disorder (option A) habitually violate the rights of others. **(pp. 412–420)**

17.19  Avoidant personality disorder can be very difficult to distinguish from which of the following disorders?

A. Social anxiety disorder.
B. Generalized anxiety disorder.
C. Panic disorder.
D. Persistent depressive disorder.
E. Autism spectrum disorder.

**The correct response is option A: Social anxiety disorder.**

Avoidant personality disorder symptoms overlap significantly with social anxiety disorder (option A). Several response options are plausible, but incorrect. Generalized anxiety disorder (option B) is accompanied by chronic anxiety but not interpersonal deficits. Panic disorder (option C) causes discrete episodes of anxious and panicky feelings but is not accompanied by social deficits, although it is often comorbid with social anxiety disorder. Persistent depressive disorder (option D) is characterized by chronic depression, and that may be accompanied by low self-esteem that can contribute to social withdrawal. Persons with autism spectrum disorder (option E) may be socially withdrawn and have social communication deficits and restrictive, repetitive patterns of behavior. **(pp. 93, 154–155, 179–182, 187, 419)**

17.20 Ebenezer Scrooge comes to your practice seeking therapy for life dissatisfaction. He spends all his time working even though he is very wealthy. A cheerless man, he is reluctant to spend his money on basic amenities such as heating during the cold winter months. He has no social life and few recreational interests. He often rejects his nephew's dinner invitations. He expresses rigid, controversial opinions, such as that donating to charity is wasteful given that his hard-earned tax dollars finance workhouses and debtors' prisons. He micromanages his sole employee, but he reserves several tasks for himself for fear that his employee is not competent to handle these necessities to his satisfaction. Which of the following is the most likely diagnosis?

A. Schizoid personality disorder.
B. Narcissistic personality disorder.
C. Obsessive-compulsive personality disorder.
D. Avoidant personality disorder.
E. Antisocial personality disorder.

**The correct response is option C: Obsessive-compulsive personality disorder.**

Charles Dickens was a remarkable observer of human behavior and foibles and captures the essence of obsessive-compulsive personality disorder in Ebenezer Scrooge, perhaps his most memorable character (option C). The disorder is characterized by uncompromising rigidity and perfectionism to the exclusion of pleasurable activities. Scrooge may have some elements of narcissistic and antisocial personality disorders (options B, E) in that he appears to lack empathy for his long-suffering assistant, Bob Cratchit. Schizoid personality disorder (option A) could be a plausible response because Scrooge is emotionally cold and detached. Yet earlier in life, as Dickens reveals, Scrooge had a rich social life and enjoyed close relationships. There is no reason to believe that Scrooge has an avoidant personality disorder (option D), because while he has a constricted social life, he does not appear to experience feelings of inadequacy or interpersonal hypersensitivity. **(pp. 409, 412, 417, 419, 421–422)**

# —CHAPTER 18—

# Psychiatric Emergencies

18.1  Aggressive behavior is associated with which of the following findings in the cerebrospinal fluid (CSF)?

A. Dopamine excess.
B. Norepinephrine excess.
C. Serotonin deficiency.
D. Acetylcholine deficiency.
E. Glutamine excess.

**The correct response is option C: Serotonin deficiency.**

At a neurophysiological level, aggressive behavior has been associated with disturbed central nervous system serotonin function. Low CSF 5-hydroxyindoleacetic acid (5-HIAA) levels are correlated with impulsive violence (option C), one of the best-replicated laboratory findings in psychiatry. (5-HIAA is a metabolite of serotonin.) It has been hypothesized that serotonin acts as the central nervous system's natural policing mechanism, helping to keep impulsive and violent behavior in check. **(p. 429)**

18.2  Which of the following is the single best predictor of future violent behavior?

A. Threats of violence.
B. Diagnosis of a severe mental illness (e.g., schizophrenia, bipolar disorder).
C. Previous psychiatric hospitalization.

D. Substance abuse history.

E. History of violence.

**The correct response is option E: History of violence.**

Although long-range predictions of violent behavior are beyond the skills of mental health professionals, they are able to predict violence in clinical settings. A patient's history of violent behavior is probably the single best predictor of future dangerousness (option E). Clinical wisdom suggests that past behavior predicts future behavior. The accuracy of predictions is improved in clinical populations that have high base rates for violence, such as patients on locked psychiatric inpatient units. That said, the importance of options A–D should not be dismissed in making a clinical assessment as well as, for example, inability to control anger, a history of impulsive behavior, paranoid ideation, and frank psychosis. **(p. 428; Table 18–1 [Clinical variables associated with violence], p. 430)**

18.3    Which of the following personality disorders is most often associated with violent behavior?

A. Paranoid personality disorder.

B. Antisocial personality disorder.

C. Schizotypal personality disorder.

D. Narcissistic personality disorder.

E. Schizoid personality disorder.

**The correct response is option B: Antisocial personality disorder.**

Cluster B ("acting-out") personality disorders such as antisocial and borderline personality disorders are associated with violent behavior (option B), a fact that is reflected by their high prevalence among incarcerated persons. **(p. 429)**

18.4    Which of the following best describes the natural history of antisocial and borderline personality disorders?

A. Patients tend to act out more as they grow older.

B. Patients tend to act out less as they grow older.

C. Patients' tendency to act out does not change.

D. Patients only tend to act out less with age if they do not have a childhood history of conduct disorder.

E. Patients only tend to act out less with age if they do not have a childhood history of fire setting or cruelty to animals.

**The correct response is option B: Patients tend to act out less as they grow older.**

With advancing age and maturity, patients with antisocial and borderline personality disorders tend to act out less often (option B), not more often (option A). A childhood history of conduct disorder is necessary to make the diagnosis of antisocial personality disorder (option D). A childhood history of fire setting and cruelty to animals increases the risk for acting-out behavior in adulthood, but there is no reason to believe that their absence will nullify the tendency for acting-out behaviors to diminish with age (option E). **(p. 429)**

18.5 A psychiatrist is called to evaluate a patient in the emergency department whose chief complaint is homicidal ideation. The psychiatrist remains calm and speaks softly. She seats herself for the interview and allows distance between herself and the patient. She is careful to always make direct eye contact and to project empathy and concern. She asks nonjudgmental questions during the interview. Which of the following behaviors displayed by the psychiatrist is *not* recommended?

A. Speaking softly.
B. Sitting during the interview because psychiatrists should stand in order to be ready to escape.
C. Projecting empathy and concern because it can seem patronizing to a violent patient.
D. Use of direct eye contact.
E. Asking nonjudgmental questions.

**The correct response is option D: Use of direct eye contact.**

Direct eye contact should be avoided when assessing potentially violent patients (option D). The clinician should speak softly, remain seated, project empathy and concern, and ask nonjudgmental questions (options A–C, E). **(p. 430)**

18.6 You are seeing a patient with schizophrenia in the emergency department. The patient acknowledges his diagnosis and reports a worsening of symptoms. He reports that he has been hearing voices that have been telling him to kill a family member, something that he does not want to do. He has been hospitalized multiple times but does not have a history of violence. The patient is pleasant and cooperative. Which of the following is the most concerning risk factor for violence?

A. Lack of insight.
B. Stated desire to hurt or kill.
C. Presence of command hallucinations.
D. Diagnosis of panic disorder.
E. History of psychiatric hospitalization.

**The correct response is option C: Presence of command hallucinations.**

The major risk factor for violence in this case is the presence of command hallucinations (option C). The patient shows some insight (option A) into his illness and does not voice a personal desire to follow through with this command (option B). Diagnosis of panic disorder and history of psychiatric hospitalization (options D, E) are not in themselves major clinical variables associated with violence. **(Table 18–1 [Clinical variables associated with violence], p. 430)**

18.7 Which of the following combinations of medications is commonly given to calm acutely agitated patients?

A. Alprazolam and diphenhydramine.
B. Chlorpromazine and clonazepam.
C. Olanzapine and lorazepam.
D. Haloperidol and lorazepam.
E. Diphenhydramine and alprazolam.

**The correct response is option D: Haloperidol and lorazepam.**

Haloperidol, 2–5 mg, and lorazepam, 1–2 mg, can be given to a patient every 30 minutes until sedation is achieved (option D). Many of the other medications are sedating, but the haloperidol-lorazepam combination has become standard practice for dealing with acute agitation. **(p. 431)**

18.8 Fill in the blank: Suicide is the _____ leading cause of death in persons between ages 15 and 24 years.

A. First.
B. Second.
C. Third.
D. Fifth.
E. Eleventh.

**The correct response is option C: Third.**

Suicide is the third leading cause of death for persons between ages 15 and 24 years (option C). It is the tenth most frequent cause of death for adults in general. **(p. 432)**

18.9 Which of the following is true regarding most people who commit suicide?

A. They usually do not tell anyone before committing suicide.
B. They may tell a friend or family member but usually do not seek medical help.
C. They usually communicate their suicidal intentions to and see physicians before they die.
D. They usually see a physician but do not usually tell their physician that they are having suicidal thoughts.
E. They usually do not have a primary care physician.

**The correct response is option C: They usually communicate their suicidal intentions to and see physicians before they die.**

Most people who commit suicide communicate their suicidal intentions to and see physicians before they die (option C). In fact, nearly two-thirds of suicidal persons communicate their suicidal intentions to others. Their communication may be as direct as reporting their plan and the date they intend to carry it out. Other communications are less obvious; for instance, a patient may say to his relatives, "You won't have to put up with me much longer." **(p. 433)**

18.10 Which of the following individuals is probably at highest risk for completing suicide?

A. 25-year-old divorced African American man.
B. 55-year-old married white woman.
C. 60-year-old widowed white man.
D. 19-year-old single African American woman.
E. 40-year-old divorced white woman.

**The correct response is option C: 60-year-old widowed white man.**

In the United States, most suicide completers tend to be older than 45 years, white, and separated, widowed, or divorced. **(p. 433; Table 18–2 [Clinical variables associated with suicide], p. 436)**

18.11 Which of the following is associated with a lower risk for suicide?

A. Major depression.
B. Male sex.
C. Hopelessness.
D. Substance use disorder.
E. African American race.

**The correct response is option E: African American race.**

Options A–D are all associated with elevated risk for completed suicide. African Americans have lower risk for suicide than whites (option E). **(Table 18–2 [Clinical variables associated with suicide], p. 436)**

18.12 Suicide is associated with which of the following CSF findings?

A. Dopamine excess.
B. Norepinephrine excess.
C. Serotonin deficiency.
D. Acetylcholine deficiency.
E. Glutamine excess.

**The correct response is option C: Serotonin deficiency.**

Low CSF levels of 5-HIAA, a serotonin metabolite, are correlated with both suicide (option C) and impulsive violence. **(p. 434)**

18.13  What is the most common method used to commit suicide in the United States?

A. Overdose.
B. Cutting.
C. Hanging.
D. Firearm.
E. Jumping.

**The correct response is option D: Firearm.**

Firearms are the most common method used to commit suicide in the United States (option D), perhaps because they are readily available and can be immediately lethal. Firearms are followed in frequency by poisoning (overdose; option A), hanging (option C), cutting (option B), jumping (option E), and other methods. **(p. 433)**

18.14  Which of the following is one of the strongest correlates of suicidal behavior, independent of psychiatric diagnosis?

A. Presence of a mental illness.
B. History of violence.
C. Recent psychiatric hospitalization.
D. Hopelessness.
E. Psychosocial stressors.

**The correct response is option D: Hopelessness.**

One of the strongest correlates of suicidal behavior is hopelessness, a finding independent of psychiatric diagnosis (option D). Most patients with mental illness do not commit suicide (option A). Options A–C and E represent categories that are overly general. **(pp. 433, 435)**

18.15  For which group of patients is suicide frequently preceded by the loss of a relationship in the past year?

A. Alcoholic persons.
B. Patients with major depressive disorder.
C. Older patients with cognitive decline.
D. Adolescents with behavior problems.
E. People with a personality disorder.

**The correct response is option A: Alcoholic persons.**

More than 50% of alcoholic persons who commit suicide have a history of relationship loss—usually of an intimate relationship—within the year before suicide (option A). **(p. 435)**

18.16 What medications are associated with lowered rates of suicide?

A. Haloperidol.
B. Lithium.
C. Clozapine.
D. Options A and B.
E. Options B and C.

**The correct response is option E: Options B and C.**

Lithium is associated with lower suicide risk (option B). Among the antipsychotics, only clozapine has been associated with lower rates of suicide (option C). Other medications, electroconvulsive therapy, and psychotherapy have not been shown to lower suicide risk. **(p. 437)**

# —CHAPTER 19—

# Legal Issues

19.1    Which of the following is a criminal and not a civil issue?

    A. Determining whether to hospitalize a patient for acute homi-cidal ideation against his or her will.

    B. Determining whether a patient with schizophrenia is capable of understanding court processes and assisting the court-appointed attorney.

    C. Potential Health Insurance Portability and Accountability Act (HIPAA) violations.

    D. Providing information about proposed treatments and alter-natives and ensuring that the patient is capable of under-standing these issues.

    E. Determining whether a psychiatrist was negligent in his pro-fessional duties after abruptly terminating a doctor-patient relationship because the patient did not promptly pay a bill.

**The correct response is option B: Determining whether a pa-tient with schizophrenia is capable of understanding court pro-cesses and assisting the court-appointed attorney.**

In the forensic world, the distinction between civil and criminal issues is fundamental. Whether a patient with schizophrenia can understand court processes and aid his or her attorney is an ex-ample of competence to stand trial, which is a criminal issue (op-tion B). The other major criminal legal issue is determining criminal responsibility. Options A and C–E represent civil issues. **(p. 440; Table 19–1 [Civil and criminal legal issues involving psychiatrists], p. 441)**

19.2 Which of the following is *not* a key criterion considered in civil commitment proceedings?

A. Mental illness.
B. Poor social support.
C. Dangerousness.
D. Inability to properly care for oneself.
E. "Grave disability."

**The correct response is option B: Poor social support.**

The major criteria in determination of cases of civil commitment are mental illness, dangerousness, and disability (sometimes referred to as "grave disability") (options A, C–E). Availability of social support is not one of the key criteria (option B), although it is an important consideration. **(p. 441)**

19.3 What level of evidence is generally required in cases of civil commitment?

A. Beyond a reasonable doubt.
B. Clear and convincing evidence.
C. Preponderance of the evidence.
D. Substantial evidence.
E. Some credible evidence.

**The correct response is option B: Clear and convincing evidence.**

The civil commitment process generally requires clear and convincing evidence (option B), a standard generally thought of as the level of proof needed for three of four reasonable people to agree. Options A and C–E represent other standards for evidence used in other legal proceedings. **(p. 442)**

19.4 Most states have provisions for

A. Involuntary inpatient treatment only.
B. Involuntary outpatient treatment only.
C. Both involuntary inpatient and involuntary outpatient treatment.
D. Neither involuntary nor voluntary outpatient treatment.
E. Voluntary outpatient treatment only.

**The correct response is option C: Both involuntary inpatient and involuntary outpatient treatment.**

Besides involuntary inpatient treatment, most states have provisions for involuntary outpatient treatment. Such treatment may be used when the patient is not quite ill enough to merit inpatient care, but he or she presents some risk of harm to self or others because of mental illness and will not voluntarily comply with outpatient treatment. **(p. 443)**

19.5   In which of the following situations is it the *least* clear cut whether patient confidentiality may be broken according to U.S. laws?

A. Reporting infectious disease such as tuberculosis or sexually transmitted infections.
B. Warning potential victims about threats made by patients.
C. Allowing access to medical charts for billing purposes.
D. Communicating with the family of a nonviolent psychiatric patient.
E. All the above are clear-cut cases in which confidentiality may be breached.

**The correct response is option D: Communicating with the family of a nonviolent psychiatric patient.**

In many instances, a psychiatrist may have good reason to want to have open communication with a patient's family because this may be in the best interest of the patient's care. However, it is not always legally clear cut whether the psychiatrist may break confidentiality in these cases (option D), although some states do have provisions to allow for this sort of communication. It is clear cut that confidentiality may be breached regarding reporting of infectious diseases and warning potential victims about threats to their person (options A, B). Insurance companies, utilization review groups, and physician peer reviewers frequently have access to medical records for billing purposes (option C). **(pp. 443–444)**

19.6   Which of the following are reasons that psychiatrists are sued for malpractice?

A. Failure to obtain informed consent.
B. Patient suicide.

C. Alleged injury from psychotropic medication.
D. Patient abandonment.
E. All the above.

**The correct response is option E: All the above.**

There are many reasons that psychiatrists are sued, and options A–D represent some of the common reasons. **(pp. 445–446)**

19.7　What percentage of physicians will face at least one malpractice suit at some point during their careers?

A. 10%.
B. 35%.
C. 50%.
D. 65%.
E. 80%.

**The correct response is option D: 65%.**

Malpractice is negligence in the conduct of one's professional duties. The number of malpractice suits filed in the United States seems to climb each year. About two-thirds of physicians will experience at least one malpractice lawsuit during their professional career (option D). The reaction among many physicians is to practice "defensive medicine," for example, ordering extra tests or refusing to treat certain patients. **(p. 445)**

19.8　According to the American Psychiatric Association, at what point does it become acceptable for a psychiatrist to have an intimate relationship with a former patient?

A. 6 months after termination of the doctor-patient relationship.
B. 1 year after termination of the doctor-patient relationship.
C. 3 years after termination of the doctor-patient relationship.
D. 10 years after termination of the doctor-patient relationship.
E. Never.

**The correct response is option E: Never.**

Sexual activity with current or former patients has become a well-publicized reason for malpractice litigation. Unlike errors in professional judgment, inappropriate sexual behavior with a patient is a voluntary act by a clinician and thus is both preventable and excluded under most malpractice insurance policies. A psychiatrist may be expelled from professional associations, have his or her license suspended or revoked, and even face criminal charges for such "boundary violations." The American Psychiatric Association has made it clear that sexual contact with current or previous patients is inappropriate and unethical. **(p. 446)**

19.9    In order to be competent to stand trial, a defendant must meet all the following criteria *except*

A. Being able to understand the nature of the charges against him or her.
B. Being able to understand the possible penalty.
C. Having been shown to have both bad behavior and blameworthy state of mind at the time of the offense.
D. Being able to understand the legal issues and procedures.
E. Being capable of working with an attorney in preparing the defense.

**The correct response is option C: Having been shown to have both bad behavior and blameworthy state of mind at the time of the offense.**

Competence to stand trial is a legal determination, not a medical one. It is determined by a judge according to national standards established by the U.S. Supreme Court in *Dusky v. United States*. To receive a fair trial, the following are required for establishing competence: a person must be able to understand the nature of the charges against him or her (option A), the possible penalty (option B), and the legal issues and procedures (option D), and he or she also must be able to work with the attorney in preparing the defense (option E). The presence of a mental illness, even a psychosis, generally does not render the defendant incompetent to stand trial. Competence to stand trial is assumed unless questioned by someone in the court. Bad behavior and blameworthy state of mind at the time of the offense (option C) are components of criminal responsibility rather than competence to stand trial. **(pp. 446–447)**

19.10 According to current U.S. laws, a crime occurs when

A. Illegal behavior occurs, regardless of the perpetrator's state of mind.
B. Illegal behavior occurs, and the perpetrator has a blameworthy state of mind.
C. A perpetrator has a blameworthy state of mind regardless of whether illegal behavior occurs.
D. Illegal behavior occurs, and the person does not have demonstrable mental illness.
E. A person with mental illness has a blameworthy state of mind.

**The correct response is option B: Illegal behavior occurs, and the perpetrator has a blameworthy state of mind.**

For a crime to occur, both bad behavior (*actus rea*) and a blameworthy state of mind (*mens rea*) must be present. A person may be so mentally ill as to lack this blameworthy state of mind by virtue of his or her disorder. In such a case, a person is said to lack criminal responsibility and is adjudicated as not guilty by reason of insanity. **(p. 447)**

19.11 Which of the following forms the basis of the insanity defense?

A. The *M'Naghten* standard.
B. The *Drummond* standard.
C. *Dusky v. United States.*
D. The *Tarasoff* rule.
E. The Peel Law.

**The correct response is option A: The *M'Naghten* standard.**

The *M'Naghten* standard established standards for determining criminal responsibility (option A). Drummond and Peel (options B, E) are names of individuals who were also involved in the M'Naghten case. The *Tarasoff* rule (option D) refers to the duty to protect. *Dusky v. United States* (option C) established standards for competency to stand trial rather than criminal responsibility. **(p. 447)**

19.12  A patient reveals to his psychiatrist that he plans to harm a neighbor. The psychiatrist is obligated to break confidentiality in order
to protect the potential victim. How shall the psychiatrist proceed?

A. Phone the neighbor to report the threat.
B. Phone the local police.
C. Ask the patient to phone the neighbor.
D. Report the threat to the local newspaper.
E. None of the above.

**The correct response is option A: Phone the neighbor to report
the threat.**

The *Tarasoff* rule refers to the duty to protect third parties from
the actions of patients in their care. On rare occasions, while
treating a patient, the patient may threaten to harm an identifiable third party. The psychiatrist has a legal responsibility to protect that third party and may break confidentiality by notifying
the threatened person and/or the police. Although the approach
to warning a third party has been debated, phoning the neighbor
directly (option A) is the best option. Some psychiatrists will do
this in the patient's presence. Phoning the local police (option B)
may be worthwhile, but the message may not reach the intended
victim. Asking the patient to phone the neighbor (option C) will
probably not lead to the patient making the phone call. Reporting
the threat to the local newspaper (option D) is not an acceptable
response. **(p. 444)**

19.13  A woman with a psychosis is charged with murder. During her
pretrial screening, her speech is disorganized such that she cannot engage in coherent dialogue with her attorneys. Which of the
following best describes her legal situation regarding the charges
against her?

A. She is competent to stand trial but not guilty by reason of in-
sanity.
B. She is not competent to stand trial and not guilty by reason of
insanity.
C. She is not competent to stand trial, and whether she is not
guilty by reason of insanity has yet to be demonstrated.
D. She is guilty but mentally ill.
E. She has diminished capacity.

**The correct response is option C: She is not competent to stand trial, and whether she is not guilty by reason of insanity has yet to be demonstrated.**

The ability to communicate with an attorney in order to prepare a defense is a component of competency to stand trial. Whether the patient has criminal responsibility has yet to be determined (option C). Guilty but mentally ill and diminished capacity (options D, E) refer to degrees of criminal responsibility implemented by some states. **(p. 447)**

# — CHAPTER 20 —

# Psychotherapy

20.1   In what form of therapy would the therapist offer praise, reassurance, and encouragement and give specific advice with the goal of helping the patient get through a difficult situation?

A. Cognitive-behavioral therapy.
B. Interpersonal psychotherapy.
C. Supportive psychotherapy.
D. Acceptance and commitment therapy.
E. Psychodynamic psychotherapy.

**The correct response is option C: Supportive psychotherapy.**

Supportive psychotherapy is the most common individual psychotherapy and is used to help patients get through difficult situations (option C). Cognitive-behavioral therapy (option A) has the goal of helping patients restructure their negative cognitions so that they can perceive reality in a less distorted way and learn to react accordingly. Interpersonal psychotherapy (option B) is a treatment for major depressive disorder and other conditions in which the therapist helps the patient identify specific problem areas that may be interfering with self-esteem and interpersonal interactions. Acceptance and commitment therapy (option D) focuses on helping individuals adapt to pain, grief, and inevitable disappointments that are part of life by developing greater psychological flexibility. In psychodynamic therapy (option E), a neutral therapist helps the patient understand the underlying dynamics that shape his or her behavior. **(pp. 450–457)**

20.2 A therapist tells a patient who is afraid of elevators to ride an elevator continuously until his or her anxiety is gone. What is this technique called?

A. In vivo exposure
B. Imaginal exposure.
C. Behavioral activation.
D. Flooding.
E. Relaxation training.

**The correct response is option D: Flooding.**

Flooding involves teaching patients to extinguish anxiety produced by a feared stimulus by placing them in continuous contact with the stimulus and helping them learn that the stimulus does not lead to feared consequences (option D). With in vivo exposure, the therapist tells a patient to enter a feared situation and use relaxation techniques while there (option A). Imaginal exposure involves having the patient imagine himself or herself in a feared situation (option B). Behavioral activation seeks to reengage patients in various activities to reverse withdrawal and isolation (option C). Relaxation training (option E) teaches patients to control their bodies and mental states through techniques such as progressive muscle relaxation. **(pp. 452–454)**

20.3 Exposure, flooding, and relaxation training are techniques used in which form of psychotherapy?

A. Cognitive-behavioral therapy.
B. Behavior therapy.
C. Acceptance and commitment therapy.
D. Psychodynamic therapy.
E. Interpersonal psychotherapy.

**The correct response is option B: Behavior therapy.**

Techniques used in behavior therapy include exposure, flooding, relaxation training, behavior modification, and behavioral activation (option B). **(pp. 452–454)**

20.4  What form of therapy has the goal of helping individuals adapt to the pain, grief, and inevitable disappointments that are part of life by developing greater psychological flexibility?

A. Supportive psychotherapy.
B. Cognitive-behavioral therapy.
C. Interpersonal psychotherapy.
D. Psychodynamic psychotherapy.
E. Acceptance and commitment therapy.

**The correct response is option E: Acceptance and commitment therapy.**

Acceptance and commitment therapy helps individuals adapt to the pain, grief, and inevitable disappointments that are part of life by promoting acceptance of what cannot be changed, while encouraging the person to cultivate the habit of committing to doing things in line with their identified hopes, values, and goals even in the face of their desire to avoid painful and troubling thoughts and emotions (option E). Supportive psychotherapy (option A) is the most common individual psychotherapy and is used to help patients get through difficult situations. Cognitive-behavioral therapy (option B) has the goal of helping patients restructure their negative cognitions so that they can perceive reality in a less distorted way and learn to react accordingly. Interpersonal psychotherapy (option C) is a treatment for major depressive disorder and other disorders in which the therapist helps the patient identify specific problem areas that may be interfering with self-esteem and interpersonal interactions. With psychodynamic therapy (option D), a neutral therapist helps the patient understand the underlying dynamics that shape his or her behavior. **(pp. 450–457)**

20.5  A therapist has a patient visualize being in an elevator to help him overcome his fear of elevators. This is an example of which of the following?

A. Relaxation training.
B. Imaginal exposure.
C. In vivo exposure.
D. Flooding.
E. Behavioral activation.

**The correct response is option B: Imaginal exposure.**

This is an example of imaginal exposure because the exposure to the feared situation—such as riding in an elevator—takes place within the patient's imagination (option B). In vivo exposure (option C) involves exposure to a real situation. Flooding (option D) involves placing patients in continuous contact with the feared stimulus. Relaxation training (option A) involves learning techniques such as deep breathing and progressive muscle relaxation to relieve anxiety. Behavioral activation (option E) is a component of behavior therapy that attempts to reengage patients in various activities to reverse withdrawal and isolation. **(pp. 452–453)**

20.6   A therapist is working with a professional musician who has depression. The patient tells the therapist that she stopped playing the guitar 2 months earlier because it no longer brings her pleasure. She previously had been playing the guitar for several hours daily. The therapist proposes that she begin playing the guitar again every day, despite her lack of interest. This is an example of which of the following?

A. Relaxation training.
B. Imaginal exposure.
C. In vivo exposure.
D. Flooding.
E. Behavioral activation.

**The correct response is option E: Behavioral activation.**

This therapist's recommendation is an example of behavioral activation (option E). The patient is instructed to engage in her previous activities with the goal of restoring her functional status as part of treatment of her depression. In turn, and consistent with behavioral theory, mood improves following restoration of important behavioral sequences in daily life. The other responses (options A–D) are components of behavior therapy. **(pp. 452–453)**

20.7   Which of the following is *not* part of Beck's cognitive triad of depression?

A. Negative view of oneself.
B. Negative view of relationships.
C. Negative view of the future.

D. Negative interpretation of experience.

E. More than one of the above.

**The correct response is option B: Negative view of relationships.**

Beck's cognitive triad of depression is a negative view of oneself, a negative view of the future, and a negative interpretation of experience (options A, C, D). Certainly, patients with depression often have a negative view of their relationships, but this is not a key part of Beck's cognitive triad (option B). **(p. 454)**

20.8   Learning to correct automatic thoughts, schemas, and distortions is a key part of which kind of therapy?

A. Behavior therapy.

B. Cognitive-behavioral therapy.

C. Interpersonal therapy.

D. Psychodynamic psychotherapy.

E. Supportive psychotherapy.

**The correct response is option B: Cognitive-behavioral therapy.**

Learning to correct automatic thoughts, schemas, and distortions is integral to cognitive-behavioral therapy (option B). Behavior therapy (option A) emphasizes correction of observable objective behavior rather than cognitions. Interpersonal therapy (option C) emphasizes improving interpersonal relationships by working on specific problem areas that may be interfering with self-esteem and interpersonal interactions. Psychodynamic psychotherapy (option D) focuses on reviewing early and current relationships via concepts derived from psychoanalysis, such as transference. Supportive psychotherapy (option E) involves providing affirmations and specific advice to help people cope with their stressors. **(pp. 450–457)**

20.9   An overzealous premedical student believes that she must get a perfect score on all of her assignments to have a chance of getting into medical school lest she be forced to spend the rest of her career working in the food service industry. This is an example of which of the following?

A. Overgeneralization.

B. Selective abstraction.

C. Dichotomous thinking.
D. Personalization.
E. Magnification and minimization.

**The correct response is option C: Dichotomous thinking.**

Dichotomous thinking is a cognitive distortion in which the patient sees things in an all-or-none way (option C). The student in this example feels that she needs to have absolutely perfect grades or she will be a failure. Overgeneralization (option A) involves making general conclusions about overall experiences and relationships based on a single instance. Selective abstraction (option B) is taking a detail out of context and using it to denigrate the entire experience. Personalization (option D) is interpreting events as reflecting on oneself when they have no relation to the individual. Magnification and minimization (option E) involve altering the significance of specific events in a way that is structured by negative interpretations. **(Table 20–4 [Cognitive distortions treated with cognitive-behavioral therapy], p. 456)**

20.10 A chess player wins three matches and loses one. He concludes that he got lucky in the three matches that he won and that he lost the other match because he is a terrible chess player. This is an example of which of the following?

A. Arbitrary inference.
B. Overgeneralization.
C. Dichotomous thinking.
D. Personalization.
E. Magnification and minimization.

**The correct response is option E: Magnification and minimization.**

The chess player is minimizing his successes, attributing them to luck, and magnifying his loss, taking it as evidence that he is a terrible player. This is magnification and minimization (option E). Arbitrary inference (option A), drawing an erroneous conclusion from an experience, is not a bad answer, but option E is better. Overgeneralization (option B) means drawing general conclusions based on a single experience. Dichotomous thinking (option C) means seeing things in an all-or-none manner. Personalization (option D) means interpreting events as reflecting on the patient when there is no relationship. **(Table 20–4 [Cognitive distortions treated with cognitive-behavioral therapy], p. 456)**

20.11 A hard-working businesswoman arrives 30 minutes late to work because of an unexpected traffic jam caused by a car accident. She berates herself for her lack of responsibility and punctuality. This is an example of which of the following?

A. Arbitrary inference.
B. Overgeneralization.
C. Dichotomous thinking.
D. Personalization.
E. Magnification and minimization.

**The correct response is option D: Personalization.**

This is an example of personalization (option D). The businesswoman blames herself for being late when she had no way to control the unexpected event. Arbitrary inference (option A) is drawing an erroneous conclusion from an experience. Overgeneralization (option B) means drawing general conclusions based on a single experience. Dichotomous thinking (option C) means seeing things in an all-or-none manner. Magnification and minimization (option E) means altering the significance of specific events in a way that is structured by negative interpretations. **(Table 20–4 [Cognitive distortions treated with cognitive-behavioral therapy], p. 456)**

20.12 What is the most important component of relationship psychotherapy?

A. The empathic and caring attitude of the therapist.
B. The neutrality of the therapist.
C. Reflection on early life experiences.
D. The correction of negative automatic thoughts and schemas.
E. Working on interpersonal disputes and deficits.

**The correct response is option A: The empathic and caring attitude of the therapist.**

The most important component of relationship psychotherapy is the empathic and caring attitude of the therapist (option A). The therapist serves as a loving and trustworthy surrogate parent who assists the patient, who is confronting unrecognized needs and unresolved drives. The therapist is more neutral but still supportive in psychodynamic therapy (option B). Reflection on early life experiences (option C) is a part of psychodynamic, insight-oriented, and relationship psychotherapy. The correction of negative automatic thoughts and schemas (option D) is part of cognitive-behavioral therapy. Interpersonal disputes and deficits (option E) are two of the four areas of concentration in interpersonal psychotherapy. **(pp. 454–457)**

20.13 One of your patients is experiencing stress and anxiety that you attribute to coping with the new responsibilities that come with parenthood. Which type of psychotherapy would be especially suited to address this sort of problem?

A. Behavior therapy.
B. Cognitive-behavioral therapy.
C. Psychodynamic psychotherapy.
D. Interpersonal therapy.
E. Supportive therapy.

**The correct response is option D: Interpersonal therapy.**

The patient is having trouble with making a role transition. Role transitions are a key domain of interpersonal therapy (option D). That said, the patient could benefit from the therapies in options A–C and E. **(pp. 450–457)**

20.14 Which of the following is *not* one of the four domains of interpersonal therapy?

A. Grief.
B. Interpersonal disputes.
C. Acceptance and commitment.
D. Role transitions.
E. Interpersonal deficits.

**The correct response is option C: Acceptance and commitment.**

Acceptance and commitment therapy is a form of therapy that targets emotional regulation (option C). Options A, B, D, and E represent the four key domains of interpersonal therapy. **(pp. 455, 457)**

20.15 A 26-year-old woman seeks treatment of her mood instability, difficult relationships, and self-harming behaviors. She is angry and irritable and says that previous therapists have not helped. She takes fluoxetine for her depression and anxiety, but it provides little symptomatic relief. She asks if there is something else you can do for her. Which of the following programs might be beneficial to her?

A. Dialectical behavior therapy (DBT).
B. Mentalization therapy.
C. Systems Training for Emotional Predictability and Problem Solving.
D. Schema-focused therapy.
E. All the above.

**The correct response is option E: All the above.**

The woman in the vignette appears to have borderline personality disorder, which is challenging to treat and responds poorly to medication. Fortunately, several evidence-based programs have been developed specifically to treat people with this condition. Perhaps the best known is DBT (option A), a program that combines group and individual therapy. DBT was developed by Marcia Linehan in the 1980s initially as a treatment for suicidal women, but borderline personality disorder is viewed as a disorder of emotional dysregulation. Options B–D are all therapies that have been developed for borderline personality disorder patients. The main barrier to treatment is that these programs may not be available. **(p. 458)**

20.16 You are seeing a 23-year-old man with schizophrenia in your office. The patient does not have any active positive symptoms of psychosis but is awkward in interpersonal interactions and has difficulty with everyday tasks (e.g., maintaining appropriate hygiene). Which form of therapy would be beneficial in order to improve this patient's functional status?

A. Behavior therapy.
B. Cognitive-behavioral therapy.

C. Psychodynamic psychotherapy.
D. Interpersonal therapy.
E. Social skills training.

**The correct response is option E: Social skills training.**

Social skills training is a specific type of psychotherapy that focuses primarily on developing abilities in relating to others and in coping with the demands of daily life, and it can substantially improve the quality of life of patients with severe mental illness such as schizophrenia (option E). Other forms of therapy (options A–D) may have some benefit for this patient, but social skills training is the modality that will best address the patient's identified deficits. **(pp. 452–457, 460)**

# —CHAPTER 21—

# Somatic Treatments

21.1  What was the world's first antipsychotic?

A. Haloperidol.
B. Thioridazine.
C. Fluphenazine.
D. Chlorpromazine.
E. Trifluoperazine.

**The correct response is option D: Chlorpromazine.**

Chlorpromazine was introduced in 1952 by the French psychiatrists Jean Delay and Pierre Deniker after they recognized that the drug had powerful calming effects on agitated psychotic patients. The trade name of chlorpromazine is Thorazine, which is easily confused with thioridazine (option B), another first-generation antipsychotic. Options A, C, and E are other first-generation antipsychotic drugs. **(p. 463)**

21.2  Compared with chlorpromazine, haloperidol

A. Has more anticholinergic side effects.
B. Is less sedating.
C. Causes fewer extrapyramidal side effects (EPS).
D. Is more likely to cause orthostatic hypotension.
E. Is associated with a much greater incidence of metabolic syndrome.

**The correct response is option B: Is less sedating.**

Haloperidol is less sedating than chlorpromazine (option B), is less likely to cause orthostatic hypotension (option D), has fewer anticholinergic side effects (option A), and is more likely to cause EPS (option C). Second-generation antipsychotics are more likely to induce a metabolic syndrome (option E). **(p. 464; Table 21–1 [Common antipsychotic agents], p. 465)**

21.3 The potency of first-generation antipsychotic drugs correlates most closely with which of the following?

A. Affinity for 5-hydroxytryptamine (serotonin) type 2A (5-HT$_{2A}$) receptors.
B. Anticholinergic activity.
C. Antihistaminic activity.
D. Dopamine 2 (D$_2$) receptor affinity.
E. Noradrenergic receptor affinity.

**The correct response is option D: Dopamine 2 (D$_2$) receptor affinity.**

The potency of first-generation antipsychotic drugs correlates with their ability to block endogenous dopamine at D$_2$ receptors (option D). Second-generation antipsychotics are weaker D$_2$ blockers but also block 5-HT$_{2A}$ receptors (option A). Central 5-HT$_{2A}$ receptor antagonism is believed to broaden the therapeutic effect of the drug while reducing the incidence of EPS associated with D$_2$ antagonists. Second-generation agents also have significant anticholinergic and antihistaminic activity (options B, C). Antipsychotics have some activity on the noradrenergic system (option E), but it does not correlate with its therapeutic potency. **(pp. 464–467)**

21.4 As a general rule, most oral antipsychotics have a half-life of approximately

A. 1 hour.
B. 4 hours.
C. 12 hours.
D. 1 day.
E. 5 days.

**The correct response is option D: 1 day.**

Nearly all antipsychotics have a half-life of 24 hours or longer and have active metabolites with longer half-lives (option D). However, depot formulations have even longer half-lives and may take 3–6 months to reach steady state. **(p. 467)**

21.5 Which of the cytochrome P450 (CYP) enzymes is involved in the metabolism of antipsychotic medications?

A. 2D6.
B. 1A2.
C. 3A4.
D. 2D6, 1A2, and 3A4.
E. Metabolism does not occur because they are renally excreted.

**The correct response is option D: 2D6, 1A2, and 3A4.**

Most first-generation antipsychotics are metabolized by the CYP enzyme subfamilies, including 2D6, 1A2, and 3A4 (option D). Because of genetic variation, 5%–10% of whites poorly metabolize medications through the CYP2D6 pathway, as do a significant proportion of African Americans. This can result in higher antipsychotic blood levels than anticipated in some patients. **(p. 467)**

21.6 You are following a 21-year-old man with schizophrenia on an inpatient psychiatric unit. After 4 weeks, he remains floridly psychotic despite increasing doses of haloperidol, administered as oral tablets. His haloperidol blood level is 1 ng/mL. What does this suggest?

A. Psychotic symptoms are refractory to treatment with haloperidol.
B. The patient is a rapid metabolizer of haloperidol.
C. The patient is not swallowing the haloperidol tablets.
D. This blood level suggests laboratory error.
E. Haloperidol blood levels do not correlate with treatment response.

**The correct response is option C: The patient is not swallowing the haloperidol tablets.**

With haloperidol, optimal response appears to be associated with serum concentrations between 5 and 15 ng/mL (option E). Because the patient in this scenario has a blood level of 1 ng/mL and continues to show significant psychosis, it is likely that he is "cheeking" his medications and spitting them out (option C). Although laboratory error (option D) is possible, it is less likely than option C. Option A is not appropriate because with such a low blood level, the psychiatrist cannot conclude that the patient's disorder is treatment refractory. There is no reason given in the vignette to suggest that the patient is a rapid metabolizer (option B). **(p. 467)**

21.7    You are following a 21-year-old man with schizophrenia who has been hospitalized for 6 weeks. The patient continues to be floridly psychotic despite increasing doses of haloperidol, administered as oral tablets. His haloperidol blood level is 15 ng/mL. What does this suggest?

A. Psychotic symptoms are refractory to treatment with haloperidol.
B. The patient is a rapid metabolizer of haloperidol.
C. The patient is not swallowing the haloperidol tablets.
D. This blood level suggests laboratory error.
E. Haloperidol blood levels do not correlate with treatment response.

**The correct response is option A: Psychotic symptoms are refractory to treatment with haloperidol.**

Many patients have a delayed response to medication, but it is worrisome that he has not had any improvement despite adequate blood levels (option A). If he were "cheeking" the tablets (option C), he would not have such a high blood level of haloperidol. Laboratory errors (option D) are always a possibility but not as likely an explanation as refractory response to treatment. There is no reason given in the vignette to suggest that the patient is a rapid metabolizer (option B). Option E is not appropriate because haloperidol blood levels are known to correlate with treatment response. **(p. 467)**

21.8    How long is an adequate trial of an antipsychotic drug?

A. 4–6 days.
B. 4–6 weeks.
C. 2–3 months.
D. 6–8 months.
E. The duration of an adequate trial depends on the specific agent.

**The correct response is option B: 4–6 weeks.**

An adequate trial of an antipsychotic should last from 4 to 6 weeks for any agent (option B). The trial can be extended if a patient shows partial response after this time interval, but a change of agent should be considered if the patient shows no response. **(pp. 467–468)**

21.9   What is the primary reason that clozapine is a second-line choice for treating psychosis?

A. Because many patients have refractory schizophrenia, clozapine is always in short supply.
B. Because clozapine can cause significant weight gain.
C. Because clozapine does not work as well as other antipsychotics for treating refractory symptoms.
D. Because clozapine can cause agranulocytosis, making it necessary for patients to have white blood cell counts checked regularly.
E. Because it takes 3–6 months to reach steady state.

**The correct response is option D: Because clozapine can cause agranulocytosis, making it necessary for patients to have white blood cell counts checked regularly.**

Clozapine is a second-line agent for treating schizophrenia because it can cause agranulocytosis and requires patients starting clozapine to have their white blood cell count checked weekly for the first 6 months, then less frequently thereafter (option D). Clozapine works better than other antipsychotics for treating refractory symptoms (option C), but it is not usually in short supply (option A). Clozapine can cause weight gain, but other antipsychotics can as well (option B). Clozapine reaches steady state as quickly as other orally administered antipsychotic drugs (option E). Depot injections such as haloperidol decanoate can take 3–6 months to reach steady state. **(pp. 134, 468–470)**

21.10   You are seeing a 21-year-old man with schizophrenia in the outpatient clinic. His psychotic symptoms have been in remission on a moderate dose of haloperidol for the past 3 years. He has been admitted to the hospital three times for acute exacerbations of his psychosis but has never engaged in dangerous behaviors. He is in school and reports that he has a good mood. The patient is interested in discontinuing antipsychotic medications, even though he has tolerated the medication well. What is your recommendation?

A. "Now would be a good time for a trial without medications."
B. "We should make sure that you remain stable for another 2 years before attempting to discontinue medications."
C. "You should take the medication for the rest of your life."
D. "Let's try a new antipsychotic medication."
E. "Let's substitute a mild antidepressant for your other symptoms such as lack of motivation."

**The correct response is option B: "We should make sure that you remain stable for another 2 years before attempting to discontinue medications."**

About 75% of stable patients taking antipsychotics will relapse within 6–24 months when taken off their medications compared with 30% of those who continue to take medications. After an initial episode of psychosis, patients should remain on medications for at least 1–2 years (option B), whereas patients with multiple episodes should continue medications for at least 5 years before attempting to discontinue medications. Patients with a history of becoming dangerous to themselves or others should remain on antipsychotics indefinitely (option C). Some schizophrenic patients will benefit from antidepressants for an accompanying depression, but the vignette does not suggest that he is depressed (option E). **(pp. 134–135, 468)**

21.11 A patient with schizophrenia is admitted to an inpatient unit for acute psychosis, agitation, and violent ideation. He has had two recent (and similar) admissions, and he readily admits to not taking prescribed aripiprazole tablets because he believes that they are poisoned. His symptoms have responded well to antipsychotics when prescribed and monitored in the hospital. Which of the following is the best long-term strategy for managing the patient's symptoms?

A. Switch to a long-acting injectable antipsychotic.
B. Restart aripiprazole.
C. Switch to clozapine.

D. Switch to haloperidol.

E. Switch to risperidone.

**The correct response is option A: Switch to a long-acting injectable antipsychotic.**

A long-acting injectable antipsychotic is the best strategy for addressing the patient's medication noncompliance (option A). It is not likely that he will continue to take oral medications after discharge given his history. Some long-acting injectables can be given monthly and others every 2 weeks. **(pp. 468–469)**

21.12 You are seeing a 35-year-old woman with schizoaffective disorder in the outpatient clinic. The patient's psychotic symptoms have been well controlled on fluphenazine for the past several years. In interview, she displays abnormal involuntary movements of her mouth and tongue of which she is not aware. The movements are most consistent with which of the following?

A. Pseudoparkinsonism.

B. Akathisia.

C. Tardive dyskinesia.

D. Acute dystonic reaction.

E. Anticholinergic side effect.

**The correct response is option C: Tardive dyskinesia.**

Tardive dyskinesia is an EPS of long-term antipsychotic use. It consists of abnormal involuntary movements, usually of the mouth and tongue, but other muscle groups can be affected (option C). Options A, B, D, and E refer to other side effects of antipsychotic medications. Valbenazine and deutetrabenazine are U.S. Food and Drug Administration (FDA) approved to treat tardive dyskinesia. **(pp. 469–470)**

21.13 A 19-year-old man recently started on haloperidol for schizophrenia comes to the clinic as a walk-in requesting to be seen urgently for "anxiety." The patient paces in the waiting room, is fidgety, and squirms in a chair during an interview. Which of the following best explains the patient's symptoms?

A. Akathisia.

B. Generalized anxiety disorder.

C. Mania.
D. Acute dystonic reaction.
E. Tardive dyskinesia.

**The correct response is option A: Akathisia.**

Akathisia is the most common form of EPS associated with antipsychotic drugs, particularly first-generation antipsychotics such as haloperidol (option A). It is characterized by subjective feelings of anxiety and tension and objective fidgetiness and agitation. Given the patient's diagnosis and that the symptoms developed shortly after he was started on an antipsychotic medication, generalized anxiety disorder (option B), mania (option C), and tardive dyskinesia (option E), none of which presents in this fashion, are unlikely. An acute dystonic reaction (option D) involves sustained muscle contractions rather than acute anxiety and does not explain the man's symptoms. **(pp. 469–470)**

21.14 A 42-year-old woman presents to the emergency department complaining of muscle stiffness. Her neck is twisted to the left, and she reports that she cannot move it. She was discharged from the inpatient psychiatric unit a day earlier after starting antipsychotic treatment for an acute psychosis. Which of the following is the best way to manage her symptoms?

A. Discontinue the antipsychotic.
B. Switch to a different antipsychotic.
C. Administer intramuscular benztropine or diphenhydramine.
D. Administer oral propranolol.
E. Administer oral clonidine.

**The correct response is option C: Administer intramuscular benztropine or diphenhydramine.**

The patient is experiencing an acute dystonic reaction induced by the antipsychotic. This usually occurs during the first 4 days of treatment and involves sustained contractions of the muscles of the neck, mouth, tongue, or occasionally other muscle groups. Patients seek immediate relief, and acute dystonic reactions typically respond within 20–30 minutes to intramuscular benztropine or diphenhydramine (option C). Although the antipsychotic could be stopped or a different antipsychotic prescribed (options A, B), these options will not provide immediate relief. Oral propranolol is effective for treating an akathisia but not an acute dystonic reaction (option D). Clonidine, an $\alpha_2$-receptor agonist, is a second-line treatment for akathisia and is not used to treat acute dystonic reactions (option E). **(pp. 469–470, 500–502)**

21.15 Which of the following is *not* an anticholinergic adverse effect of antipsychotics?

A. Diarrhea.
B. Urinary retention.
C. Blurry vision.
D. Dry mouth.
E. Exacerbation of narrow-angle glaucoma.

**The correct response is option A: Diarrhea.**

Constipation, not diarrhea, is an anticholinergic side effect of antipsychotics (option A). Options B–E are typical anticholinergic side effects that tend to occur commonly with low-potency agents such as chlorpromazine. **(p. 470)**

21.16 Regular monitoring of body mass index (BMI), blood pressure, fasting glucose, and lipid panels is recommended for patients who are taking which of the following?

A. Haloperidol.
B. Risperidone.
C. Venlafaxine.
D. Sertraline.
E. Nortriptyline.

**The correct response is option B: Risperidone.**

Because second-generation antipsychotics (e.g., risperidone) are linked with metabolic abnormalities, it is recommended that patients have baseline measures of BMI, waist circumference, blood pressure, and fasting glucose and lipid panels (option B). Afterward, blood pressure, lipid panels, and fasting glucose should be followed up every 3 months, then annually. Options A and C–E are medications from other classes without standard guidelines for measuring these parameters. **(p. 471)**

21.17 A 45-year-old woman who takes haloperidol for her schizophrenia is admitted to a medical unit for rigidity, high fever, and mental status changes. Laboratory tests show elevated creatinine phosphokinase and liver enzymes. What is the most important aspect of acute care for this patient?

A. Start dantrolene.
B. Start bromocriptine.
C. Start electroconvulsive therapy (ECT).
D. Stop haloperidol and provide supportive care.
E. Transfer to psychiatric inpatient unit.

**The correct response is option D: Stop haloperidol and provide supportive care.**

Neuroleptic malignant syndrome (NMS) is a medical emergency. NMS is a rare, idiosyncratic side effect of antipsychotics, typically first-generation antipsychotics such as haloperidol. The most important aspect of treatment is to stop the offending drug and provide supportive care (option D). Although dantrolene (option A), bromocriptine (option B), and ECT (option C) have all been used to treat NMS, the drug must first be discontinued. NMS should not be managed on a psychiatric inpatient unit (option E). **(pp. 471, 565)**

21.18 You are treating a 35-year-old man for a major depressive disorder and narcissistic personality disorder. He demands that he receive the most effective antidepressant available. What do you do?

A. Prescribe levomilnacipran because it is one of the newer antidepressants.
B. Prescribe escitalopram because it is a standard selective serotonin reuptake inhibitor (SSRI).
C. Prescribe venlafaxine because of its dual action in targeting norepinephrine and serotonin neurotransmission.
D. Advise him that antidepressants are—for the most part—equally effective.
E. Recommend psychotherapy to address his underlying narcissism.

**The correct response is option D: Advise him that antidepressants are—for the most part—equally effective.**

Antidepressants typically have a 65%–70% response rate within 4–6 weeks versus 25%–40% for a placebo, and, with minor exceptions, all are equally effective (option D). **(p. 473)**

21.19  Which type of depression is expected to respond best to an antidepressant?

A. Persistent depressive disorder (dysthymia).
B. Atypical depression.
C. Major depressive disorder with comorbid hypochondriasis.
D. Major depressive disorder with comorbid somatic symptom disorder.
E. Major depressive disorder with melancholic features.

**The correct response is option E: Major depressive disorder with melancholic features.**

Patients with major depressive disorder with melancholic features (e.g., diurnal variation, psychomotor agitation or retardation, terminal insomnia, pervasive anhedonia) might respond better to antidepressants than do nonmelancholic depressed patients (option E). Atypical depression might preferentially respond to monoamine oxidase inhibitors (MAOIs; option B). Persistent depressive disorder, a chronic form of depression, also can be treated with antidepressants, but the treatment results are not as robust as those seen in other forms of depression (option A). Major depressive disorder with comorbid hypochondriasis or somatic symptom disorder are not recognized depressive subtypes (options C, D). **(pp. 158–159, 473, 485–486)**

21.20  Which SSRI has the longest half-life?

A. Fluoxetine.
B. Sertraline.
C. Citalopram.
D. Escitalopram.
E. Paroxetine.

**The correct response is option A: Fluoxetine.**

Fluoxetine has a half-life around 2–3 days (option A), but its major metabolite, norfluoxetine, has a half-life of 4–16 days. The other SSRIs have half-lives ranging from 15 to 35 hours. All are well absorbed and reach peak plasma levels within 4–8 hours. **(p. 477)**

21.21 Which of the following is *not* a typical SSRI adverse effect?

A. Loose bowel movements.
B. Anxiety.
C. Sexual dysfunction.
D. Nausea.
E. Orthostatic hypotension.

**The correct response is option E: Orthostatic hypotension.**

Options A–D are typical side effects of SSRIs except for orthostatic hypotension (option E), which is associated with tricyclic antidepressants and MAOIs. **(pp. 477–478)**

21.22 You prescribe citalopram to a 28-year-old man for obsessive-compulsive disorder. At follow-up, he reports that his symptoms have greatly improved, but he has developed delayed ejaculation that interferes with a new relationship. Which pharmacological strategy has *not* been recommended to address this problem?

A. Switch to bupropion.
B. Add bupropion to the citalopram.
C. Switch to duloxetine.
D. Take lorazepam prior to sexual activity.
E. Take sildenafil prior to sexual activity.

**The correct response is option D: Take lorazepam prior to sexual activity.**

The development of an SSRI-induced sexual disorder creates a dilemma for the psychiatrist, particularly if the patient has responded well to the drug. The best option is to stop the offending drug, but this may not be desirable, particularly if the patient—as in this vignette—has obsessive-compulsive disorder, which responds preferentially to these agents. All the strategies in options A–C and E have been used and may help, except for taking lorazepam (option D). Lorazepam can help with hyperstimulation caused by an SSRI or with the SSRI discontinuation syndrome. **(p. 477)**

21.23 A 55-year-old woman is brought to the emergency department with an altered mental status, flushing, diaphoresis, and myoclonic jerks. She was recently started on a third antidepressant for treatment-refractory depression. Which of the following is the most likely diagnosis?

A. Catatonia.
B. Serotonin syndrome.
C. NMS.
D. SSRI discontinuation syndrome.
E. Acute dystonic reaction.

**The correct response is option B: Serotonin syndrome.**

Serotonin syndrome presents with symptoms of lethargy, restlessness, mental confusion, flushing, diaphoresis, tremor, and myoclonic jerks (option B). If untreated, serotonin syndrome can progress to hyperthermia, hypertonicity, rhabdomyolysis, renal failure, and death. Patients who are concurrently taking two or more drugs that boost central nervous system serotonin levels are at higher risk. Coadministration of an MAOI and an SSRI could trigger a serotonin syndrome. Symptoms of serotonin discontinuation syndrome include nausea, headache, vivid dreams, irritability, and dizziness (option D). NMS (option C) is characterized by rigidity, high fever, and elevated levels of creatine phosphokinase and occurs in patients taking antipsychotic medication. Catatonia and acute dystonic reactions (options A, E) are not characterized by flushing, diaphoresis, or myoclonic jerks. **(pp. 471, 478)**

21.24 Which antidepressant is contraindicated for a 45-year-old man with epilepsy?

A. Venlafaxine.
B. Mirtazapine.
C. Trazodone.
D. Bupropion.
E. Desvenlafaxine.

**The correct response is option D: Bupropion.**

Bupropion can cause seizures, particularly at dosages greater than 450 mg/day. Thus, it is contraindicated in patients with a seizure disorder or an eating disorder (option D). Patients with an eating disorder (e.g., bulimia nervosa) may have a lower seizure threshold from an electrolyte disturbance. Seizure is the major risk of bupropion overdose. **(pp. 479–480)**

21.25 Which of the following patients is a good candidate for a trial of duloxetine?

A. A 37-year-old woman with a history of multiple recent overdose attempts.
B. A 60-year-old man with chronic depression and alcoholism.
C. A 20-year-old man with depression, posttraumatic stress disorder, and insomnia.
D. A 54-year-old woman with depression partially controlled by an MAOI.
E. A 48-year-old man with major depressive disorder and neuropathic pain from diabetes mellitus.

**The correct response is option E: A 48-year-old man with major depressive disorder and neuropathic pain from diabetes mellitus.**

Duloxetine is FDA approved to treat major depressive disorder, generalized anxiety disorder, diabetic neuropathic pain, and fibromyalgia (option E). It can be fatal in doses as low as 1,000 mg and thus should be avoided in patients at high risk for overdose (option A), and it can cause hepatotoxicity, so duloxetine should be avoided in patients who drink heavily (option B) or have liver disease. As with most antidepressants, it should not be combined with an MAOI (option D) because of the risk of serotonin syndrome. Mirtazapine is a better choice for a patient with major depression, posttraumatic stress disorder, and insomnia, because it can help with sleep (option C). **(pp. 480–481)**

21.26 Which of the following antidepressants is the best choice for a 30-year-old man with a first episode of major depressive disorder with melancholic features including insomnia and weight loss?

A. Citalopram.
B. Bupropion.
C. Duloxetine.
D. Mirtazapine.
E. Venlafaxine.

**The correct response is option D: Mirtazapine.**

The medications in options A–C and E would not be contraindicated for this patient; however, mirtazapine (option D) would be a particularly good choice because it can help with sleep disturbance, and as a side effect, it increases appetite, which can lead to weight gain. **(pp. 473–482)**

21.27  Which of the following antidepressants is widely used off-label to treat insomnia?

A. Venlafaxine.
B. Duloxetine.
C. Trazodone.
D. Phenelzine.
E. Sertraline.

**The correct response is option C: Trazodone.**

Trazodone is widely used off-label to treat insomnia because it is very sedating (option C). **(pp. 278, 481–482)**

21.28  A 35-year-old man who has treatment-refractory depression presents to the emergency department because of a prolonged painful erection. The patient has been taking multiple psychotropic medications to treat his disorder, including sertraline, bupropion, buspirone, trazodone, and lithium. Which medication is most likely to have caused his condition?

A. Sertraline.
B. Bupropion.
C. Buspirone.
D. Trazodone.
E. Lithium.

**The correct response is option D: Trazodone.**

Priapism, a prolonged painful erection, is an uncommon side effect of trazodone (option D). Men who are prescribed trazodone should be warned about this potential side effect and instructed to seek immediate medical attention should it occur. **(pp. 481–482)**

21.29 What is the mechanism of action of the antidepressant vilazodone?

A. It selectively inhibits reuptake of serotonin.
B. It inhibits reuptake of both serotonin and norepinephrine.
C. It is a dopamine $D_2$ receptor antagonist.
D. It is a serotonin reuptake inhibitor and 5-HT$_{1A}$ receptor partial agonist.
E. It blocks 5-HT$_2$ receptors and weakly inhibits serotonin reuptake.

**The correct response is option D: It is a serotonin reuptake inhibitor and 5-HT$_{1A}$ receptor partial agonist.**

Vilazodone is a serotonin reuptake inhibitor and 5-HT$_{1A}$ receptor partial agonist (option D). Vilazodone is not a conventional SSRI or serotonin-norepinephrine reuptake inhibitor (SNRI; options A, B), and it does not block $D_2$ receptors (option C). **(p. 482)**

21.30 Which of the following tricyclic antidepressants has an established therapeutic blood level range?

A. Amitriptyline.
B. Nortriptyline.
C. Doxepin.
D. Clomipramine.
E. Protriptyline.

**The correct response is option B: Nortriptyline.**

The therapeutic blood level range of nortriptyline is 50–150 ng/ mL (option B). Desipramine and imipramine also have established therapeutic ranges. That said, there is no reason to routinely obtain plasma levels, particularly when the patient is doing well. Blood levels are helpful in cases of drug overdose and also may be useful when evaluating a patient's failure to respond adequately, significant symptoms of toxicity, or suspected noncompliance; in establishing a therapeutic window; and in setting dosage levels for a patient with significant cardiac or other medical disease (when it is desirable to keep the blood level at the lower range of the therapeutic value). **(pp. 483–484)**

21.31 Why are MAOIs not more widely used to treat depression?

A. Because of the required long washout period when transitioning a patient to or from an MAOI to avoid serotonin syndrome.
B. Because a hypertensive crisis could result if an MAOI is combined with foods that contain tyramine.
C. Because they are potent α-adrenergic blockers and can cause orthostatic hypotension.
D. Because patients prescribed MAOIs should carry a list of prohibited foods, wear a medical bracelet indicating that they take an MAOI, and carry a 10-mg tablet of nifedipine with them at all times.
E. All the above.

**The correct response is option E: All the above.**

All of these are reasons that MAOIs are not commonly used (option E). Although MAOIs are effective antidepressants, especially for those with an atypical depression, it is uncommon for patients to be prescribed an MAOI as a first choice. **(pp. 485–487)**

21.32 What is a reasonable length for an adequate trial of an antidepressant?

A. 3–5 days.
B. 3–5 weeks.
C. 1–2 months.
D. 3–4 months.
E. It depends on the agent.

**The correct response is option C: 1–2 months.**

Antidepressant trials should last 1–2 months (option C). If a patient does not respond at 4 weeks on the target dosage, options to consider are increasing the dose or switching to a different antidepressant. **(p. 488)**

21.33 A 25-year-old man with a well-established diagnosis of bipolar I disorder presents to the emergency department, having been brought in by the police for disruptive behavior. He has not been sleeping for the past 3 days, and he believes that he is Jesus Christ. He is very agitated, and you believe that he is potentially dangerous. Which of the following medications would be most effective in calming him while in the emergency department?

A. Lithium.
B. Valproate.
C. Lamotrigine.
D. Haloperidol.
E. Carbamazepine.

**The correct response is option D: Haloperidol.**

Mood-stabilizing medications such as lithium or carbamazepine take 5–7 days to have a noticeable effect (options A, E). The patient would benefit from prompt initiation of a mood stabilizer to treat his mania, but an antipsychotic such as haloperidol with or without a benzodiazepine can provide immediate sedation and tranquilization (option D). **(pp. 468, 490–494)**

21.34 Which of the following medications has been shown to reduce suicidal behavior?

A. Valproate.
B. Lithium.
C. Carbamazepine.
D. Lamotrigine.
E. Alprazolam.

**The correct response is option B: Lithium.**

Lithium carbonate is one of the few medications shown to reduce suicidal behaviors (option B), but care should be taken because lithium can be dangerous in overdose. **(p. 490)**

21.35 Which of the following is *not* an appropriate use of lithium?

A. Prophylaxis of manic episodes in bipolar I patients.
B. Reducing the severity of manic episodes.
C. Adjunctive treatment to prevent recurrences of depression in patients with unipolar major depressive disorder.
D. Achieving rapid sedation of an acutely agitated manic patient.
E. Prophylaxis of depressive episodes in patients with a bipolar disorder.

The correct response is option D: Achieving rapid sedation of an acutely agitated manic patient.

Lithium is a remarkable drug that can prevent and moderate mood episodes in bipolar patients (options A, B, E) and can also help to prevent recurrence of depression in patients with unipolar depression (option C). It can be used to treat mood episodes in those with schizoaffective disorder. It is sometimes used to treat aggressive behavior, but an antipsychotic or a benzodiazepine is best for rapid sedation of an agitated patient (option D). (pp. 488, 490)

21.36 When is the best time to check a lithium blood level?

A. 8 hours after the last dose for a manic patient and 18 hours after the last dose for a euthymic patient.
B. 12 hours after the last dose.
C. 8 hours after the last dose.
D. 18 hours after the last dose.
E. Accurate lithium levels can be obtained at any time because the elimination half-life of lithium is 36 hours.

The correct response is option B: 12 hours after the last dose.

Lithium levels should be checked 12 hours after the last dose (option B). Manic patients clear lithium more quickly than do euthymic patients, but the standard rule is to check the level 12 hours after the last dose whether the patient is manic, euthymic, or depressed. (p. 490)

21.37 Which mood-stabilizing agent does *not* undergo mostly hepatic metabolism?

A. Valproate.
B. Lamotrigine.
C. Lithium.
D. Carbamazepine.
E. None of the above.

The correct response is option C: Lithium.

Lithium is renally excreted and not metabolized (option C). The other medications (options A, B, and D) all undergo hepatic metabolism. (pp. 490–495)

21.38 Which mood-stabilizing agent can in rare cases cause Stevens-Johnson syndrome?

A. Valproate.
B. Lamotrigine.
C. Lithium.
D. Carbamazepine.
E. Aripiprazole.

**The correct response is option B: Lamotrigine.**

In rare cases, lamotrigine can cause potentially life-threatening Stevens-Johnson syndrome and toxic epidermal necrolysis (option B). It should not be mixed with valproate, because combination therapy increases the risk. **(p. 495)**

21.39 For which of the following cases is lamotrigine monotherapy most appropriate?

A. A patient with bipolar I disorder and a history of multiple hospitalizations for mania and a history of nonresponse to lithium.
B. A patient with bipolar I disorder with a history of multiple hospitalizations for mania and a history of response to lithium.
C. A patient with bipolar I disorder who presents with irritable mania.
D. A patient with bipolar I disorder with mixed mania and depression.
E. A patient with bipolar I disorder with several severe depressive episodes and infrequent manic episodes.

**The correct response is option E: A patient with bipolar I disorder with several severe depressive episodes and infrequent manic episodes.**

Lamotrigine appears to be most effective in delaying the time to occurrence of depressive episodes and may be effective in the treatment of acute depressive episodes as well (option E). Bipolar I disorder patients with multiple hospitalizations for mania and a history of nonresponse to lithium (option A), patients with irritable mania (option C), or patients in a mixed episode (option D) are good candidates for valproate. Those with multiple hospitalizations for mania and a history of response to lithium (option B) are good candidates for lithium. **(pp. 490, 493, 495)**

21.40 Which patient with bipolar I disorder is a good candidate for carbamazepine therapy?

A. A patient with irritable mania who has not responded to lithium.
B. A patient in a mixed episode.
C. A patient with more than four mood episodes per year who has not responded to lithium.
D. A patient with mostly depressed episodes and mild infrequent hypomanic episodes.
E. None of the above.

**The correct response is option C: A patient with more than four mood episodes per year who has not responded to lithium.**

Carbamazepine might be more effective in patients who cycle rapidly (i.e., patients who have more than four mood episodes per year) and who do not respond to lithium (option C). Patients with irritable mania or mixed episodes (options A, B) may respond better to valproate. Lamotrigine would be a good choice for a patient with mostly depressive episodes and mild infrequent hypomanic episodes (option D). **(pp. 493–495)**

21.41 Which neurotransmitter is intimately involved in the mechanism of action for benzodiazepines?

A. Glutamate.
B. Norepinephrine.
C. Gabapentin.
D. γ-Aminobutyric acid (GABA).
E. Serotonin.

**The correct response is option D: γ-Aminobutyric acid (GABA).**

Benzodiazepines are believed to exert their effects by binding to specific benzodiazepine receptors in the brain. The receptors are intimately linked to receptors for GABA, a major inhibitory neurotransmitter (option D). By binding to benzodiazepine receptors, the drugs potentiate the actions of GABA, leading to a direct anxiolytic effect on the limbic system. Gabapentin, of course, is a drug and not a neurotransmitter (option C). **(pp. 69–70, 496)**

21.42 Benzodiazepines are remarkably versatile drugs. These medications are used to treat all of the following *except*

A. Seizure disorders.
B. Anxiety.
C. Alcohol withdrawal.
D. Sleep disorders.
E. Major depressive disorder.

**The correct response is option E: Major depressive disorder.**

Benzodiazepines are useful for the treatment of generalized anxiety disorder, especially when severe (option B). Many patients benefit when their anxiety is acute and problematic; these medications generally should be given for short periods (e.g., weeks or months). Patients with mild anxiety may not need medication and can be successfully managed with behavioral interventions (e.g., progressive muscle relaxation). These drugs may be useful in treating major depressive disorder, but they have no demonstrated antidepressant effect, and their use is mainly for treating those with an anxious form of depression along with an antidepressant (option E). **(pp. 496–498)**

21.43 Which of the following medications has an FDA indication for the treatment of generalized anxiety disorder?

A. Buspirone.
B. Bupropion.
C. Alprazolam.
D. Aripiprazole.
E. None of the above.

**The correct response is option A: Buspirone.**

Buspirone is FDA approved for the treatment of generalized anxiety disorder (option A). The antidepressant bupropion (option B) has no role in treating anxiety, whereas aripiprazole (option D) is used to treat psychoses. Alprazolam (option C) has an indication to treat panic disorder but is not recommended to treat generalized anxiety disorder, except perhaps on a short-term basis as with the other benzodiazepines. **(pp. 469, 479, 497, 499)**

21.44 Extrapyramidal syndromes have been treated with all of the following medications *except*

A. Propranolol.
B. Diphenhydramine.
C. Amantadine.
D. Benztropine.
E. Trazodone.

**The correct response is option E: Trazodone.**

The choice of drug depends on the syndrome. Pseudoparkinsonism can be treated with amantadine or benztropine (options C, D). An acute dystonic reaction can be treated with intramuscular diphenhydramine (option B). An akathisia can be treated with propranolol (option A). Trazodone (option E) is not used to treat any of these syndromes. **(pp. 469–470, 500–502)**

21.45 Which of the following conditions represents an absolute contraindication to administering ECT?

A. Recent myocardial infarction.
B. Unstable coronary artery disease.
C. Space-occupying brain lesions.
D. Venous thrombosis.
E. Chronically low platelet count.

**The correct response is option C: Space-occupying brain lesions.**

Relative contraindications include recent (i.e., within 1 month) myocardial infarction (option A), unstable coronary artery disease (option B), uncompensated congestive heart failure, uncontrolled hypertensive cardiovascular disease, venous thrombosis (option D), and chronically low platelet count (option E). Space-occupying brain lesions and other causes of increased intracranial pressure, such as recent intracerebral hemorrhage, unstable aneurysms, or vascular malformations, are the only absolute contraindications to ECT (option C). **(pp. 503–504)**

21.46 A 36-year-old woman is receiving ECT for treatment of her major depressive disorder. What should she be told about possible adverse effects of the treatment?

A. She might have permanent memory loss that will be most dense around the time of treatment.
B. She will have no memory loss because the psychiatrist will use unilateral lead placement.
C. She will have permanent memory loss that will mainly involve new memories following the conclusion of the treatment.
D. She will have no memory loss because the psychiatrist will use the minimal amount of electricity needed to be therapeutic.
E. None of the above.

**The correct response is option A: She might have permanent memory loss that will be most dense around the time of treatment.**

The most troublesome long-term effect of ECT is memory loss. Because ECT disrupts new memories that have not been incorporated into long-term memory stores, ECT can cause anterograde and retrograde amnesia that is most dense around the time of treatment (option A). The anterograde component usually clears quickly, but the retrograde amnesia can extend back to months before treatment. Not all patients experience memory loss, and unilateral electrode placement, modification of the pulse wave, and the use of low dosages of electricity help minimize any loss that occurs (options B, D). They do not prevent memory loss from occurring, however. Patients must be told that permanent memory loss can occur. **(p. 506)**